Health Matters ist ein neu entwickeltes Lehrwerk speziell für medizinische Fach-angestellte im Berufsschulunterricht, die sich mit Patienten oder Kunden auf Englisch in Standardsituationen austauschen müssen. Das einbändige Lehrwerk setzt Englischkenntnisse voraus, die der Stufe A 2 des Europäischen Referenz-rahmens *(Common European Framework of Reference)* entsprechen.

Health Matters enthält 10 Units, in denen handlungsorientiert alltägliche Gege-benheiten und aktuelle Themen aus unterschiedlichen Bereichen einer Arztpraxis aufgegriffen werden. Landeskundliche Informationen über Großbritannien und über die USA werden auch vermittelt. Der Schwerpunkt liegt auf dem dialogischen Austausch in typischen Berufssituationen. Dabei wird die Sprachkompetenz an-hand zahlreicher Hörverständnis- und Sprechübungen, die von rein funktionalen Dialogen bis zu freien Diskussionen reichen, geschult. Anhand motivierender Aufgaben werden Hemmungen, sich in der Fremdsprache auszudrücken, abge-baut.

Die Grammatik in *Health Matters* ist auf das Wesentliche begrenzt. Grundlegende Strukturen werden in den Units im situativen Kontext vermittelt. Weitaus wichtiger ist jedoch die Erweiterung des berufsrelevanten Wortschatzes und das Erlernen feststehender Redewendungen, die als Rüstzeug für eine flüssige, effektive beruf-liche Kommunikation dienen.

Jede Unit enthält mindestens eine Seite mit *Extra Material* für leistungsstärkere Lernende. Das Thema der jeweiligen Unit wird anhand von anspruchsvolleren Texten und durch Hörverständnisübungen ausgebaut.

Im Anhang finden Sie die Transkripte der Hörverständnistexte sowie Auflistungen zu Zahlen, Daten und Uhrzeiten und Redewendungen für Telefonate. Abgerundet wird das Lehrwerk mit chronologischen und alphabetischen Wörterverzeichnissen sowie einer Grundwortschatzliste, die etwa 370 Wörter enthält, die für die Arbeit mit *Health Matters* als bekannt vorausgesetzt werden.

Der Verlag, der Autor und die Beraterinnen wünschen Ihnen viel Erfolg und Freude bei der Arbeit mit *Health Matters*.

Symbolerklärungen:

⊙ Hörverständnistext auf der Audio-CD

✏ schriftliche Übung

◯◯ Partnerarbeit

Contents

At reception

1 At reception

Gareth Jones is British but he lives in Germany. He is at Dr Müller's surgery, where Kerstin Vogt works as a medical assistant.

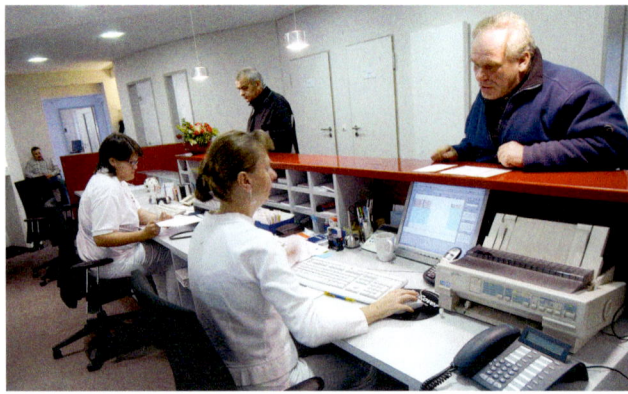

T2 Read the dialogue and then listen to it on the CD.

Kerstin	Guten Tag.
Gareth	Ah, hello. Can you speak English?
Kerstin	Yes, can I help you?
Gareth	Yes. My name's Jones. Mr Gareth Jones. I've got an appointment.
Kerstin	Mr Jones ... Ah, yes, the appointment was for ten thirty. But don't worry.

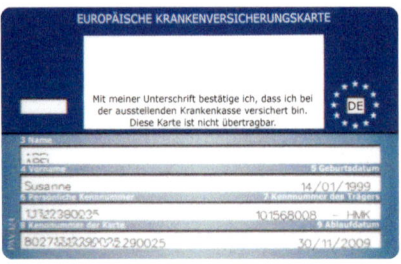

Gareth Oh, I am sorry. What time is it?

Kerstin It's twenty to eleven, but we aren't very busy today. We can fit you in.

Gareth Oh good. Thank you. Sorry.

Kerstin It's OK. Have you got your health insurance card with you?

Gareth Yes, I have. Here it is.

Kerstin And have you got ten euros for the surgery charge, please?

Gareth Yes, here you are.

Kerstin Thank you. And here's your receipt.

Gareth Thanks.

Kerstin You're welcome. Please take a seat in the waiting room.

Gareth OK. Thank you.

Are these statements true or false? Correct the false statements.

1 Gareth can speak German.
2 He has got an appointment at the surgery.
3 His appointment is for 10.40 a.m.
4 The surgery is busy today.
5 Gareth hasn't got his insurance card.
6 He can't pay the 10 euros.
7 The doctor can't see him immediately.

CULTURE *Please, thank you* and *sorry*

- British people use politenesses such as **please** and **thank you** a lot.
- They also say **sorry** very often if they inconvenience someone.
- When you give someone something and they say thank you, the correct response is **You're welcome**, and **not Please**.

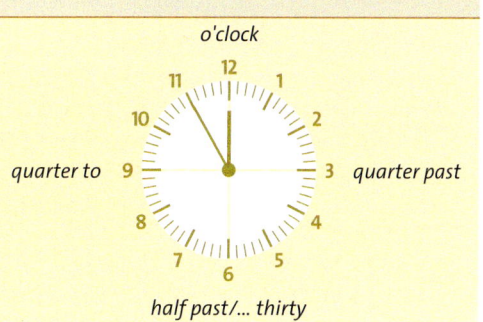
2 Telling the time

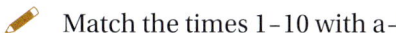 Match the times 1–10 with a–j.

1	twenty past ten	a	10:15
2	eleven o'clock	b	11:30
3	half past eleven	c	16:50
4	ten fifteen	d	10:20
5	eighteen fifteen	e	11:00
6	twenty to eleven	f	11:20
7	quarter to eleven	g	18:15
8	half past ten	h	10:30
9	eleven twenty	i	10:40
10	sixteen fifty	j	10:45

■ Auf Deutsch bedeuten *half past ten, half ten* und *ten thirty* alle **halb elf**.

■ Die Zeitangabe *o'clock* wird nur bei einer vollen Stunde benutzt, z. B. *six o'clock* = sechs Uhr.

■ Bei Zeitangaben, die nicht durch 5 teilbar sind, sollte man *minutes* verwenden.
  6:03 = *three minutes past six*
  7:13 = *thirteen minutes past seven*
  11:53 = *seven minutes to twelve*

3 What time is it?

T3 Listen to the phone calls and choose the correct appointment times.

1 10:30 / 11:30   2 4:50 / 4:15   3 12:10 / 11:50   4 8:45 / 9:15   5 8:30 / 9:30

4 Making appointments

T4 Listen to the four phone calls and write the names of the callers and the times of their appointments in an exercise book.

5 What's in the appointment book?

Work with a partner. Use the information and the phrases from exercises 3 and 4 to make dialogues.

WEDNESDAY	THURSDAY
8.35 Mr Wright	8.35 Ms Williams
9.15 Mrs Randall	12.20 Mr Graham

1 **I'm** fine, you**'re** fine, but Tom **isn't**.
2 **Is** your appointment for today or tomorrow? – It**'s** for today.
3 **Are** you in pain? – Yes, I **am**./No, **I'm not**.
4 **I've got** my receipt, but I **haven't got** my prescription.
5 **Has** she **got** her health insurance card with her? – Yes, she **has**./No, she **hasn't**.
6 **Have** you **got** your receipt for the surgery charge? – Yes, I **have**./No, I **haven't**.

be	■ Im Präsens hat das Verb drei Formen: *am, is, are.* (1, 2, 3).
	■ Die Kurzformen werden oft bei positiven Aussagen benutzt. (1, 2) Aber bei positiven Kurzantworten wird die Langform benutzt. (3)
	■ Die negativen Formen sind *am not, isn't, aren't.* (1)
	■ Bei Fragen wird das Verb an den Satzanfang gestellt. (2, 3)
have got	■ Im Präsens gibt es zwei Formen: *has got, have got* (oft zu *'ve* abgekürzt). Bei positiven Kurzantworten wird die Langform benutzt. Alle Kurzantworten sind ohne *got.*(5, 6)
	■ Die negativen Formen sind *hasn't got, haven't got.* (4)
	■ Bei Fragen wird *has* oder *have* an den Satzanfang gestellt.

6 Practice

Complete the sentences with the correct form of the verbs.
Write three more sentences.

1 The appointment … (be) for 8:45 on Thursday.
2 We … (not / be) very busy today.
3 … (be) Mr Bell in the waiting room?
4 I … (be) sorry, but you … (be) too late for your appointment.
5 I'm sorry but I … (not / have got) an appointment.

6 … (she/have got) her insurance card with her?
7 … (you/have got) ten euros?
8 Dr Thomas … (not/have got) the results of your blood test yet.
9 …
10 …
11 …

7 Spelling names

Listen to the names and choose the correct spelling.

1 a) Gawlinski   b) Gelinski   c) Gawlinka
2 a) Tunchi   b) Tuncay   c) Toonshy
3 a) Kusnetzof   b) Kasnestof   c) Kuznetsov
4 a) Yildirim   b) Yedilim   c) Yidrilm
5 a) Wizocksi   b) Wysocki   c) Wiysoke
6 a) Leigh   b) Leegh   c) Liegh

Work with a partner. Spell your names to each other.

8 Dealing with a new patient

Candy Donnelly is Australian but lives in Germany. She phones Dr Müller's surgery to make a first appointment.

Look at the box below. What does Kerstin say?

Kerstin Arztpraxis Müller. Guten Tag. Sie sprechen mit Frau Vogt.

Candy Oh hello, can you speak English?

Kerstin (1) …

Candy Oh good. Can I make an appointment, please?

Kerstin (2) …

Candy Yes, it is.

Kerstin (3) …

Candy It's Candy Donnelly.
That's D-O-double N-E-double L-Y.

Kerstin (4) …

Candy It's Kellinghusenstraße 32.

Kerstin (5) …

Candy It's 14171 Berlin.

Kerstin (6) …

Candy It's 030 89552.

Kerstin (7) …

Candy Yes, I have.

Kerstin (8) …

Candy Yes, Friday morning, please.
Can I have an early appointment?

Kerstin (9) …

Candy Yes, that's a good time. Thanks.

Kerstin (10) …

Candy That's no problem. I can come a bit early.

Kerstin Good. Thank you. So, see you on Friday. Goodbye.

> **CULTURE** Health care
>
> In the UK a doctor who works in a health centre and not in a hospital is called a General Practitioner (GP). You must be registered with a GP in order to receive health care. So when British people move house, they have to register with a new GP. You may find British patients ask to register with a doctor in Germany, too.

Work with a partner and practise similar dialogues with other names, addresses and telephone numbers.

Kerstin

a Yes I can. Can I help you?

b And the postcode, please?

c And your address, please Ms Donnelly?

d That's great. Can you bring it with you, please? Now we need to make a first appointment. Is there any day or time you would like?

e 14171. Thank you. And your telephone number?

f Is this your first appointment with our practice?

g Good. So that's Friday 18 June at twenty five to nine. Can you come fifteen minutes early, please as you need to complete a medical history form.

h Right, early. Let's have a look. Is 8.35 OK?

i Then I need to take some details first. So, can I have your full name, please?

j That's 030 89552. And have you got a health insurance card?

9 A record file

Below is Candy Donnelly's patient record file on Kerstin's computer. Copy it into your exercise book. Then read the dialogue again and write down the missing information.

Vorname: [   ]   Familienname: [   ]

Straße: [   ]   Hausnummer: [   ]   PLZ: [   ]   Stadt: [   ]

Versichertenkarte: [ja]

Datum des Termins: [18. Juni]   Tag: [   ]   Zeit: [   ]

10 Taking personal details

Copy the patient record file into your exercise book again. Then work with a partner to make a dialogue and complete the record file. Use the dialogue in exercise 8 as a model.

11 A new patient

Work with a partner. A new patient walks into your practice. It's his/her first appointment. Role play a dialogue.

Medical assistant	Patient
Begrüßen Sie die neue Patientin/den neuen Patienten und fragen Sie, ob Sie helfen können.	
	Fragen Sie die/den MFA*, ob sie/er Englisch kann.
Sagen Sie, dass Sie es können und fragen, ob sie/er einen Termin hat.	
	Sagen Sie Nein, und dass Sie das erste Mal zu diesem Arzt/dieser Ärztin gehen.
Fragen Sie nach dem Namen der Patientin/des Patienten.	
	Nennen Sie Ihren Namen.
Fragen Sie nach den nötigen persön- lichen Daten. Überprüfen Sie die Schreibweisen.	
	Geben Sie Ihre persönlichen Daten an.
Fragen Sie, wann der Patient/die Patientin gerne einen Termin hätte.	
	Machen Sie Ihren ersten Termin aus.
Bestätigen Sie den Termin und verab- schieden Sie sich.	
	Bedanken Sie sich bei der/dem MFA und verabschieden Sie sich.

*MFA = Medizinische/r Fachangestellte/r

Extra material

1 Medical receptionist training in the UK

Your boss knows you are learning English and gives you this leaflet about medical receptionist training in the United Kingdom. Read the text and note the important points about the qualifications and training. Then summarize the differences between Germany and the UK.

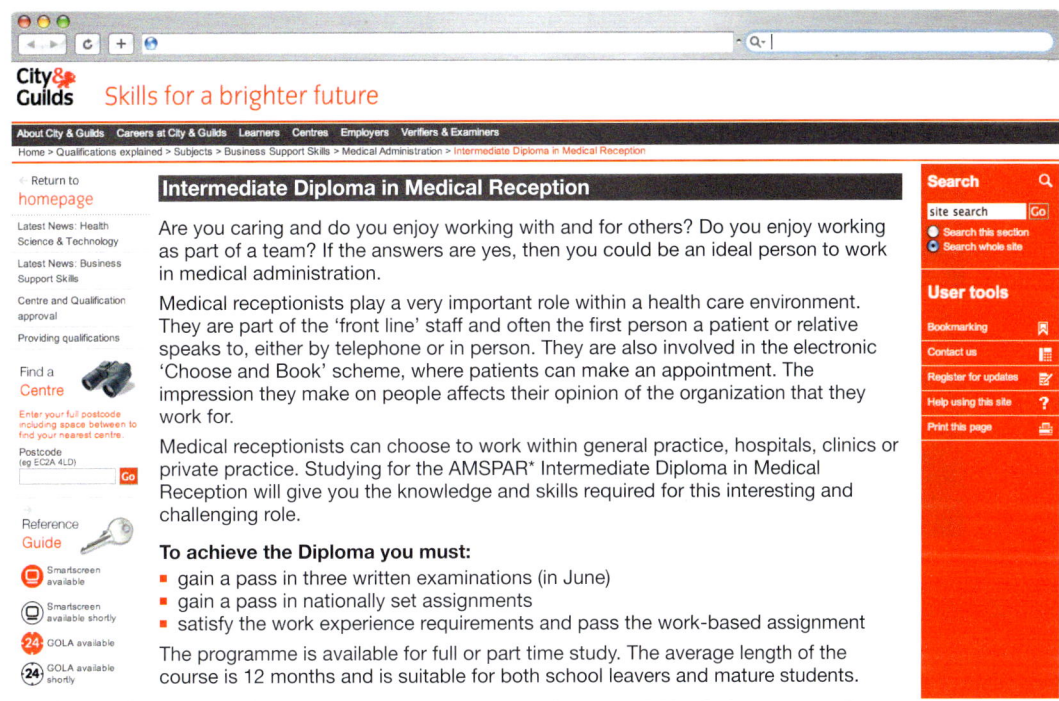

* AMSPAR: The Association of Medical Secretaries, Practice Managers, Administrators and Receptionists

2 Working with words

Match the words (1–8) with the definitions (a–h).

1	caring	a)	people who work for an organisation
2	staff	b)	thinking about what other people need or want
3	relative	c)	what you think about something
4	involved in	d)	piece of work given as part of a job
5	impression	e)	member of your family
6	opinion	f)	part of
7	required	g)	feeling you have about something or someone
8	assignment	h)	needed

1 The practice

T6 ⊙ Listen to the CD about people in a typical health centre. Match the people and the activities.

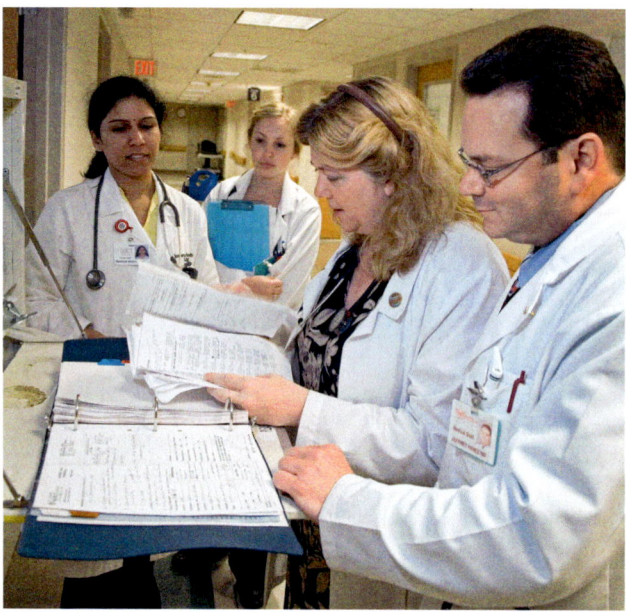

People: 1 receptionist
2 general practitioner (GP)
3 nurse 4 radiologist
5 paediatrician 6 physio-
therapist 7 gynaecologist

Activities: a) make
appointments b) take
X-rays c) do check-ups
for women d) assist the
doctor e) help with joints
and movement f) specia-
lize in treating children
g) diagnose general
health problems

2 Work with a partner

∞ Work with a partner. Look at the rooms in the health centre and say what happens in each room.

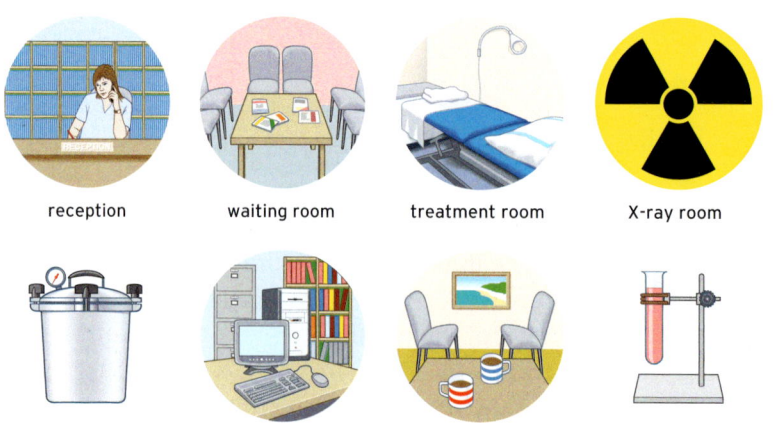

reception

waiting room

treatment room

X-ray room

sterilization room

office

staffroom

lab(oratory)

At reception, the
receptionist makes
appointments.

In the
waiting room,
patients ...

3 The medical receptionist

Read the information and answer the questions below.

Medical Receptionist

Job Description: Medical Receptionist

Pleasantown Community Health has a job opening for the following position: medical receptionist. Full time. E-mail to info@pleasantownhealth.org

Skills:

- Warm outgoing personality
- Ability to work in a supportive manner with persons of all backgrounds
- Excellent telephone skills
- Ability to work well under pressure
- Ability to work accurately and efficiently
- Must have computer knowledge, Microsoft Excel, and Word experience a must, 40 WPM*

(*= words per minute)

Duties include:

- Greet patients; be polite and helpful to the public
- Respect privacy and dignity of patients at all times
- Provide professional telephone services
- Register patients and help them to complete forms
- Make appointments for patients
- Collect fees and make online payments
- Order forms and office supplies for the front desk
- Close the building at the end of each working day; turn off or unplug appliances and machines
- Get the front desk and reception area ready for business at the start of each working day
- Take part in staff and educational meetings

1 Which are the most important skills? Rank them in order of importance.
2 Which of the skills do you think you can learn through training?
3 Look at the duties and put them in order of how often a medical receptionist must do them.
4 Are there any duties that you would add to the list?

> **CULTURE** surgery personnel
>
> In the UK, administrative staff are not trained or legally allowed to do clinical duties. Doctors can only be assisted by qualified nurses. In some states in the USA, practitioner nurses are allowed to treat patients if a doctor is present.

4 The duties of a medical receptionist

Which verbs (1–8) go with the nouns (a–h)?

1 respect	5 collect	a) appointments	e) a building
2 register	6 order	b) privacy	f) meetings
3 provide	7 close	c) fees	g) patients
4 make	8 take part in	d) services	h) forms

5 Practice

Use the information below to make complete sentences.

1. the receptionist/register/patients
   Example: The receptionist registers patients.
2. the nurse/collect/fees?
3. the GP/not make/appointments
4. I/not take/X-rays
5. the physiotherapist/not diagnose/ general health problems
6. a good receptionist/work/well under pressure
7. receptionists/need/excellent telephone skills
8. we/not keep/paper records
9. Dr Henderson/visit/her patients?
10. who/make/ the tea/in your office?
11. most patients/read/one of the magazines/in the waiting room
12. the nurse/keep/medical supplies/in this room
13. nobody/enter/the practice/without registering at reception
14. young children/not usually like/ injections

6 A GP's surgery

Describe these photos from a British medical practice.

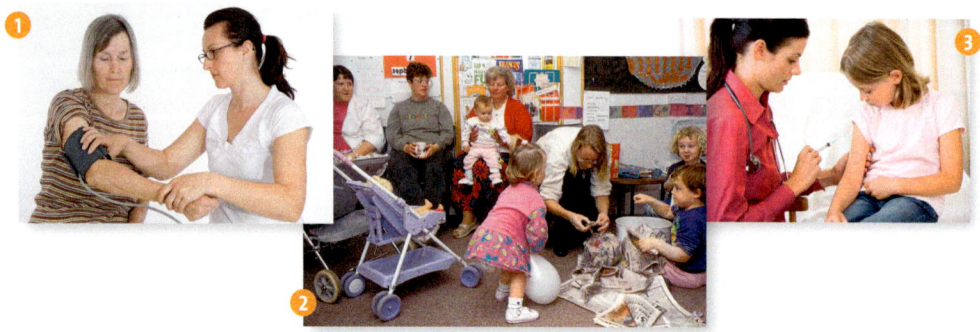

7 Describing jobs

Work with a partner. Tell your partner which of these jobs you do at work.

Start like this:

> A I make appointments.
> What about you?

> B I make appointments,
> but I don't ...

Describing jobs
- I make appointments.
- I don't take X-rays.
- As part of my duties I ...
- I'm (not) responsible for ...
- I sometimes have to ...

8 Reception and office equipment

Match these words to the illustrations below.

appointment book | appointment cards | calendar | card reader port | cash box |
printer/scanner | date stamp | fax machine | filing cabinet | inkpad | label printer |
memo pad | paper clips | scissors | stapler | suspended pocket file

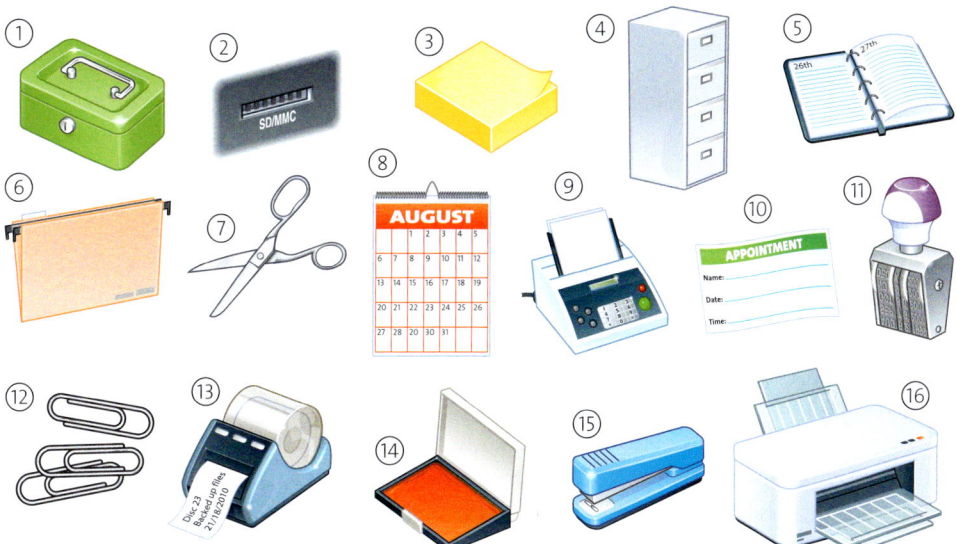

9 Working with words

Work with a partner. Use the words in the box to describe what each of the things from exercise 8 is used for.

> You store files in a ...

> You use a stapler to ...

> We don't use a ...

keep records/cash | store files | write notes | ink a date stamp | make appointments | check the date | file documents/letters | fix documents together | print documents/labels | read medical insurance cards | stamp the date | send faxes | cut things | attach cards to paper

10 Giving directions

T7 Look at the plan of the health centre. Listen to the receptionists and match the rooms to the numbers. The patients are in the waiting room.

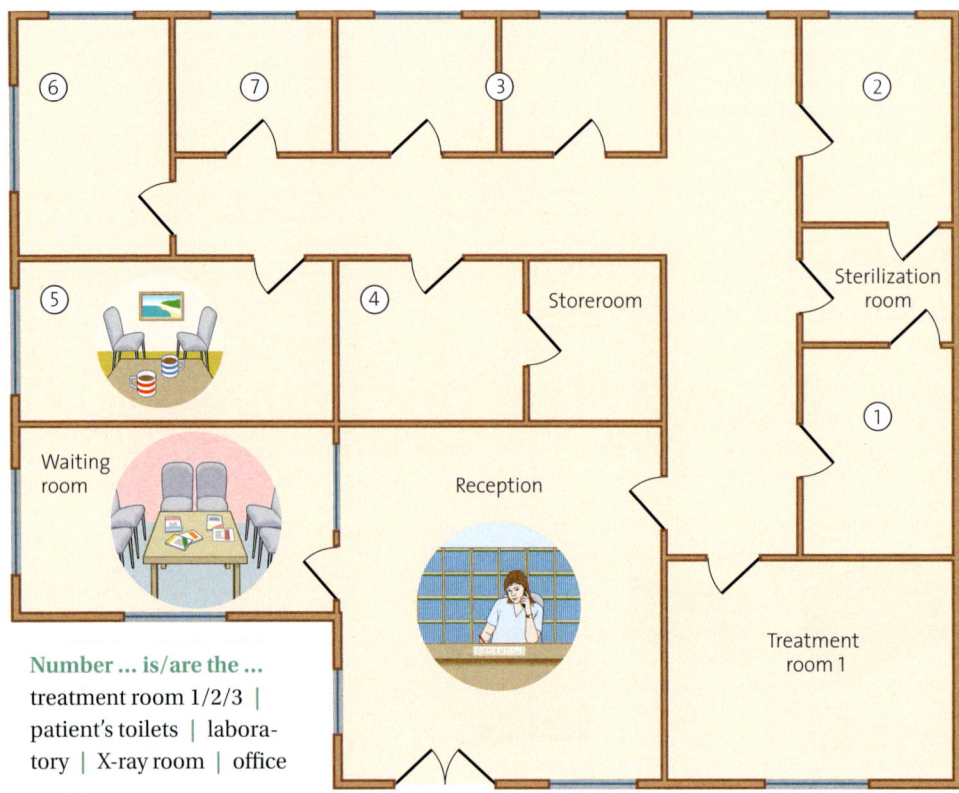

Number ... is/are the ...
treatment room 1/2/3 |
patient's toilets | labora-
tory | X-ray room | office

11 Activity

Work with a partner. Draw a plan of the practice where you work and label reception and one other room. Next to the plan, write the names of the other rooms in the practice. Give the plan to your partner. Then help each other label the plans by asking for and giving directions. Always start at reception.

Giving directions

Excuse me, where is/are the ... ?
Go straight on and then turn left/right.
Go down/along the corridor.
Go up/down the stairs.
Go through the doors and ...
It's just here in front of you.
It's (the first/second) on the left/right.
It's next to/between/opposite the ...

Where's the waiting room, please?

Excuse me, please. Can you tell me where the ... is?

It's ...

Extra material

1 Basic personal information

You have a foreign visitor in your surgery. You need the following information:

Vorname | Familienname | Adresse in Deutschland | Geburtsdatum | Telefonnummer | Handynummer | Name der Versicherung | Krankheiten

✏ Write a list of questions in English.

2 Medical history

✏ Translate these questions from a medical questionnaire into English for a foreign visitor to your practice. Use a dictionary and words from the box below.

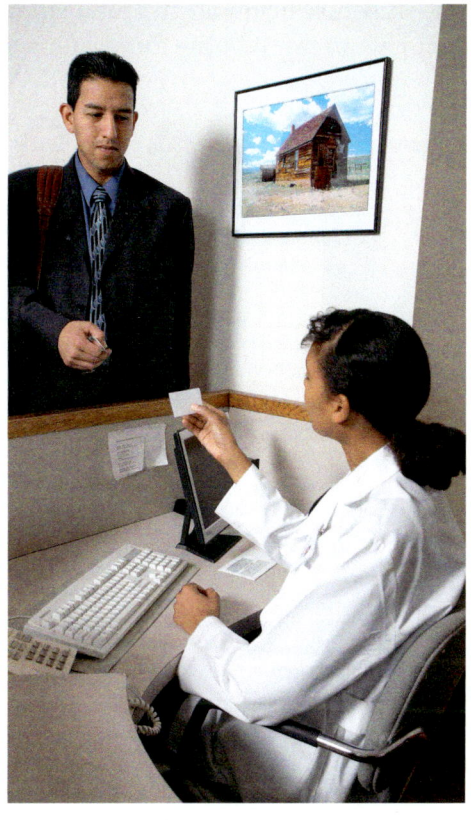

1 Sind Sie zur Zeit in ärztlicher Behandlung?
2 Hatten Sie jemals nach Einnahme von Medikamenten oder nach Spritzen oder Betäubungsmitteln eine allergische Reaktion?
3 Nehmen Sie zur Zeit Medikamente? Wenn ja, welche?
4 Sind Sie schwanger?
5 Sind Sie HIV-positiv?
6 Wann war Ihr letzter Besuch in einer Arztpraxis?
7 Haben Sie im Moment irgendwelche gesundheitliche Probleme?
8 Haben Sie Hepatitis B?
9 Werden Sie während einer ärztlichen Behandlung ängstlich oder nervös?

medical treatment | allergic reaction | drugs | injections | tablets | medicine | pregnant | HIV positive | health problems | hepatitis B | anxious

T8 ◎ Listen to the CD and hear how a nurse translated these questions.

3 Describing symptoms

1 Waiting to see the doctor

The six people below are in waiting rooms at different health centres. Read what they have to say. Who are they waiting to see?

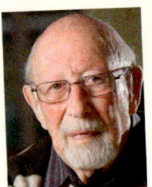

Harry Taylor

Eight weeks ago I fell down some stairs and broke my leg. It was a very bad break, so now I have to learn to walk again without crutches. I come here almost every day.

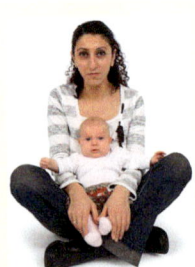

Birgül and Erkan Yildiz

I'm here with my little boy, Erkan. Our GP thought he might have asthma but he wasn't sure so he sent us here. I hope the doctor can find out what's wrong with him.

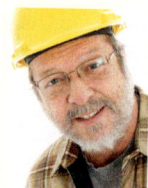

Ron Jarvis

Well, I'm a bit deaf at the moment, so I went to see the doctor last week and he told me it was just a problem with wax. So, I've got an appointment today to have my ears syringed.

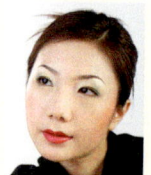

Cindy Wong

I keep getting migraines, so I went to my GP but she didn't know what was wrong. So, she sent me here to get some scans of my head.

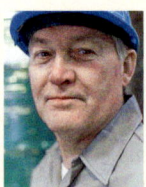

Andrew Carter

Well, I cut my arm while re-pairing a bike and it looked like a bad cut. This is the nearest health centre. It's really close by, so I walked here straight away.

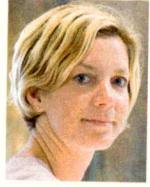

Karolina Bartolski

I'm here because I received a letter asking me to come for a smear test. It's only a routine test but I think it's a really good idea to have regular check-ups.

general practitioner (GP) | gynaecologist | nurse | paediatrician | physiotherapist | radiologist

... is waiting for ...

2 What do they do?

 Complete the sentences.

1 A ... keeps patient records and helps the doctor.
2 A ... specializes in children's illnesses.
3 A ... helps patients to exercise their joints and muscles.
4 A ... specializes in women's health problems.
5 A ... is a non-specialist doctor.

3 Working with words

 Look again at what the six patients said and write down all the verbs that are in the simple past tense. Then make a table in your exercise book like the one below.

Simple past	Infinitive form	German
had	*have*	*haben*

4 Practice

 In your exercise book, complete the sentences with the correct form of the simple past.

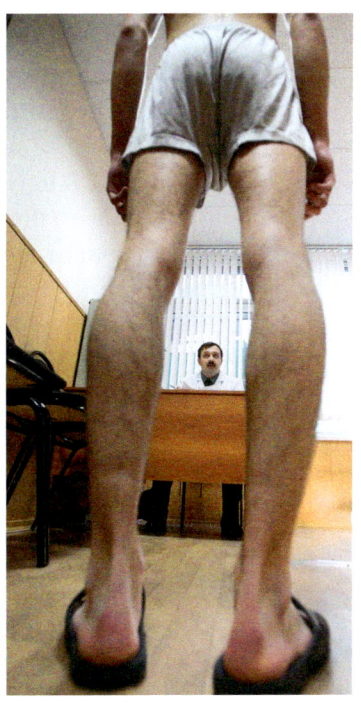

1 The doctor (tell) me I had a chest infection.
2 I (not/see) the doctor last week.
3 I (make) an appointment for you on Thursday at 9 am.
4 (you/see) the doctor yesterday?
5 The patient (have to) wait for an hour to see the doctor.
6 I (not can/get) an appointment yesterday.
7 The antibiotics (not/stop) the infection.
8 (you/take) your medicine yesterday?
9 I (receive) a letter from my GP last week.
10 My GP (not/know) what was wrong with me.
11 She (think) it was a good idea to have a check-up.
12 They (not/have) any appointments on Friday.
13 When (you/get) the letter?
14 He (break) his leg last week playing football.

5 Seeing the nurse

T9 Complete the dialogue with the simple past form of the verbs. Be careful of negatives and questions. Then listen to the CD to check your answers.

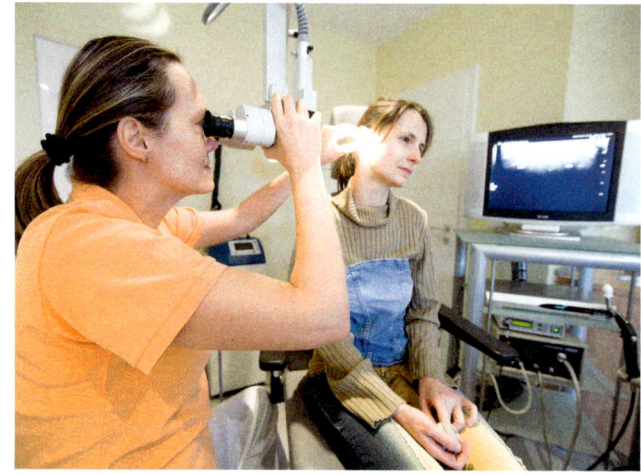

Sandra Hello, good morning Mr Jarvis. My name's Sandra Waterman. How are you today?

Ron Very well, thanks.

Sandra Is this your first visit to our practice?

Ron Yes, it is. I ... (move[1]) to the town three months ago.

Sandra Oh really? And where ... you ... (live[2]) before?

Ron In a small village called Shepton, about 6 miles away.

Sandra Oh, I know Shepton very well. Now can you hold this tray for me under your ear? That's great, thanks. And who ... (be[3]) your GP there?

Ron I ... (go[4]) to Doctor Wheeler at the Maltings Health Centre.

Sandra Oh yes, Dr Wheeler's very nice. I ... (live[5]) in Shepton for five years, but I ... (not/work[6]) at the Maltings.

Ron Where ... you ... (work[7])?

Sandra I ... (work[8]) here. Now I'm going to start syringing your ear. Tell me if it hurts at all, OK? Right here we go. I ... (begin[9]) working here twenty years ago.

Ron That's a long time! ... you always ... (want[10]) to be a nurse?

Sandra Yes, I think so. I ... (know[11]) I wanted to be a nurse when I ... (be[12]) still at school. This ... (be[13]) the first job I ... (apply[14]) for when I ... (leave[15]) school. Is this comfortable for you? It isn't painful at all?

Ron No, it's fine. I think I can hear better already!

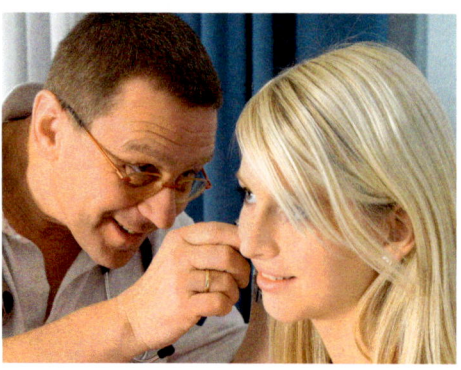

FACTFILE Medical acronyms	
ENT	Ears, nose and throat
ECG	An electrocardiograph is a machine that measures the electrical changes in your heart.
EEG	An electroencephalograph is a machine that measures electrical activity in the brain.
EMG	An electromyograph measures muscle activity.

6 The ear

Read the text and match the highlighted words to the parts of the ear in the diagram.

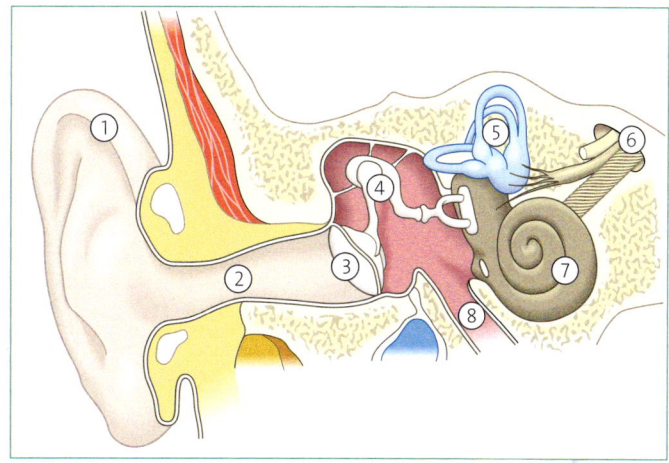

Well, first of all you have the outer ear, which begins with the ear flap. This is made of soft cartilage and is on the very outside of the ear. This channels sound waves into the external ear canal and then on to the eardrum, which separates the outer ear from the middle ear. Here the sound waves are turned into vibrations which are then amplified by the ossicles – a chain of three tiny bones, the hammer (malleus), the anvil (incus) and the stirrup (stapes). These vibrations go to the inner ear, where they are turned into signals by the cochlea and then sent to the brain by the auditory nerve. The other important parts of the inner ear are the semi-circular canals, which are fluid-filled canals that help control balance and the Eustachian tube, which connects the middle ear to the throat and keeps the pressure the same on both sides of the ear drum. This is what makes your ear 'pop' when you're on a plane!

The … is number …

7 The nose, mouth and throat

T 10 Listen to a GP talking to a class of trainee nurses about the nose, mouth and throat. Make notes in your exercise book under the following headings.

nasal passage | olfactory nerves | throat | windpipe (trachea) | palate | tongue | gullet (oesophagus)

Then use your notes and the following diagram. Name the parts and explain their function.

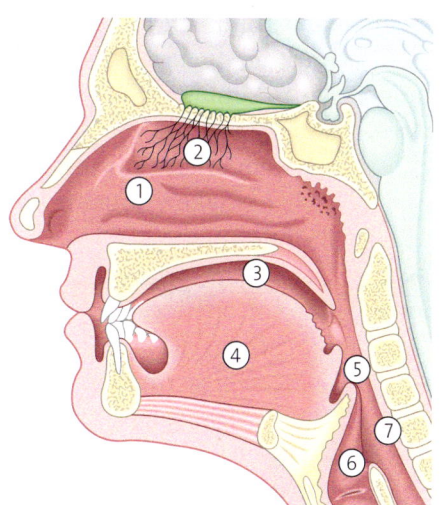

8 Working with words

Which parts of the ear, nose and mouth do you use when you taste, smell and hear?

9 Making a diagnosis

Bekri Ozalan goes to see Dr Müller with a sore throat.

 Copy the table below into your exercise books. Then read the text and complete the notes.

Patient:	Mr Bekri Ozalan
Symptoms:	
Diagnosis:	
Treatment:	

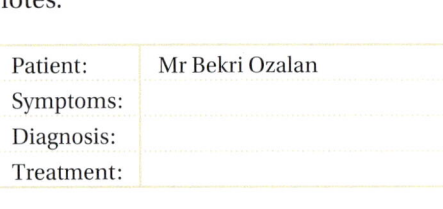

Dr Müller	Good morning Mr Ozalan. Please come in. Now, what's the problem?
Bekri	My throat is very sore and I'm not feeling very well.
Dr Müller	OK, let's have a look. Can you please put your head back and open your mouth nice and wide? Thank you. Hmm. When did your throat start feeling sore?
Bekri	About two days ago. It's really sore. I'm also having trouble swallowing.
Dr Müller	Uh huh. Can I take a quick look in your ears for a moment, please? Right, that looks OK. Now I just need to put this thermometer in your ear to take your temperature. There we go. Is that OK?
Bekri	Yes, that's OK.
Dr Müller	Right, your temperature is a little high. I just need to check your glands now. Hmm, they also feel a bit swollen. Are you having any problems breathing at all?
Bekri	No, breathing is OK, but I can't sleep very well and I feel tired all the time.
Dr Müller	Well Mr Ozalan, you have a temperature, your glands are a little swollen and your tonsils are also inflamed, so I think you probably have tonsillitis. I'd like to take a throat swab and send it to a lab to find out what caused the infection.
Bekri	OK.
Dr Müller	Can you open wide, please so I can take a swab? That's it. Thank you. I'll send this to the lab for tests. I'm going to prescribe some anti-biotics. Drink plenty of fluids, get some rest and come back in two days. I'll write you a sick note. OK?
Bekri	Yes, thank you doctor.

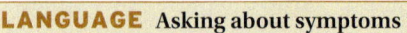

LANGUAGE Asking about symptoms

Could you tell me what's wrong?
What seems to be the problem?
Do you have/Have you got ...?
Does your neck/back/... hurt/ache?

10 Working with words

✎ Match the verbs with the nouns.

1	take	4	send	a	for tests	d	fluids
2	check	5	prescribe	b	temperature	e	glands
3	cause	6	drink	c	antibiotics	f	an infection

11 What seems to be the problem?

✎ These people are waiting to see Dr Scott. Write their names in an exercise book.

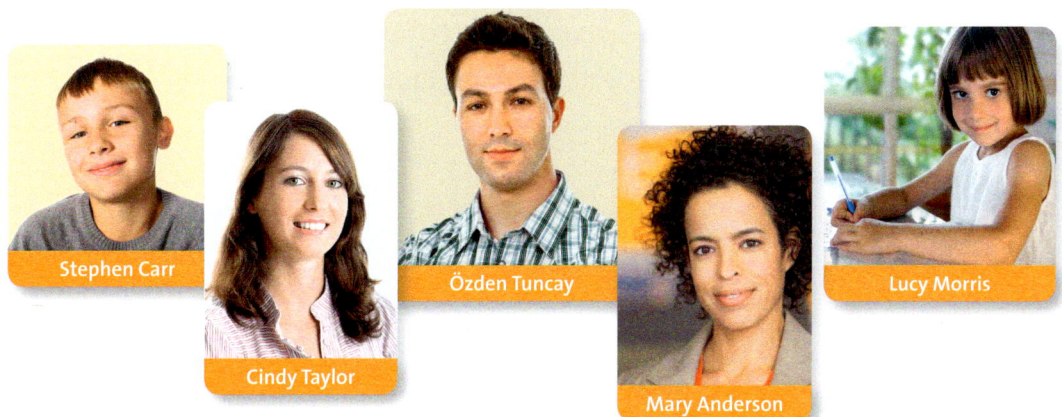

Stephen Carr

Cindy Taylor

Özden Tuncay

Mary Anderson

Lucy Morris

T11 ⊙ Now listen to these patients or their parents talking to Dr Scott. Write down their symptoms.

12 Your diagnosis

◯◯ Work with a partner and discuss each of the patients from exercise 11 and their symptoms. What is your diagnosis?

I think ... has got ...
- a cold.
- food poisoning.
- the flu. (Formal: influenza)
- an ear infection.
- (the) measles.

I agree (with you/your diagnosis).

I disagree. He/She could have ...

Yes, I think so too.

The symptoms for ... are similar.

FACTFILE Medical specialists and non-specialists

GP	General Practitioner is the name for a local doctor in the UK. A GP works for the National Health Service (NHS).
Cardiologist	A doctor who studies or treats heart diseases.
Consultant	A senior doctor who has completed all his or her training and is on a specialist register.

13 Examining the patient

T 12 Dr Grant is now ready to see Andrew Carter. Listen and note down the details.

Work with a partner and take turns asking and answering questions.

When			cut his arm?
Where	did	Mr Carter	treat him?
What		Dr Grant	give him?
How			...?

14 Working with words

Copy and complete the table with the correct form of the words.

	verb	noun
1	diagnose	...
2	...	examination
3	treat	...
4	cut	...
5	consult	...
6	stitch	...
7	...	look
8	...	dressing

① cut

② blister

③ scratches

④ bruises

⑤ rash

LANGUAGE Describing symptoms

I have/I've got
- an earache/a backache/a headache
- a sore throat
- chest/back/stomach pains
- a pain in my ...
- (a) 1/2/3/4/5 on my wrist/...

I keep coughing/sneezing/vomiting.
I have trouble sleeping/breathing/keeping food down/...
My joints/feet/head ache(s).

15 Describing symptoms

Work with a partner. One student thinks of a medical problem and describes the typical symptoms. The other guesses what it is by asking questions.

Have you got a sore throat?   *No, I haven't.*
Have you got a temperature?   *Yes, I have.*
Do your joints ache?   *Yes, they do.*

1 Women and heart disease

Read the website article about heart disease and answer the questions below.

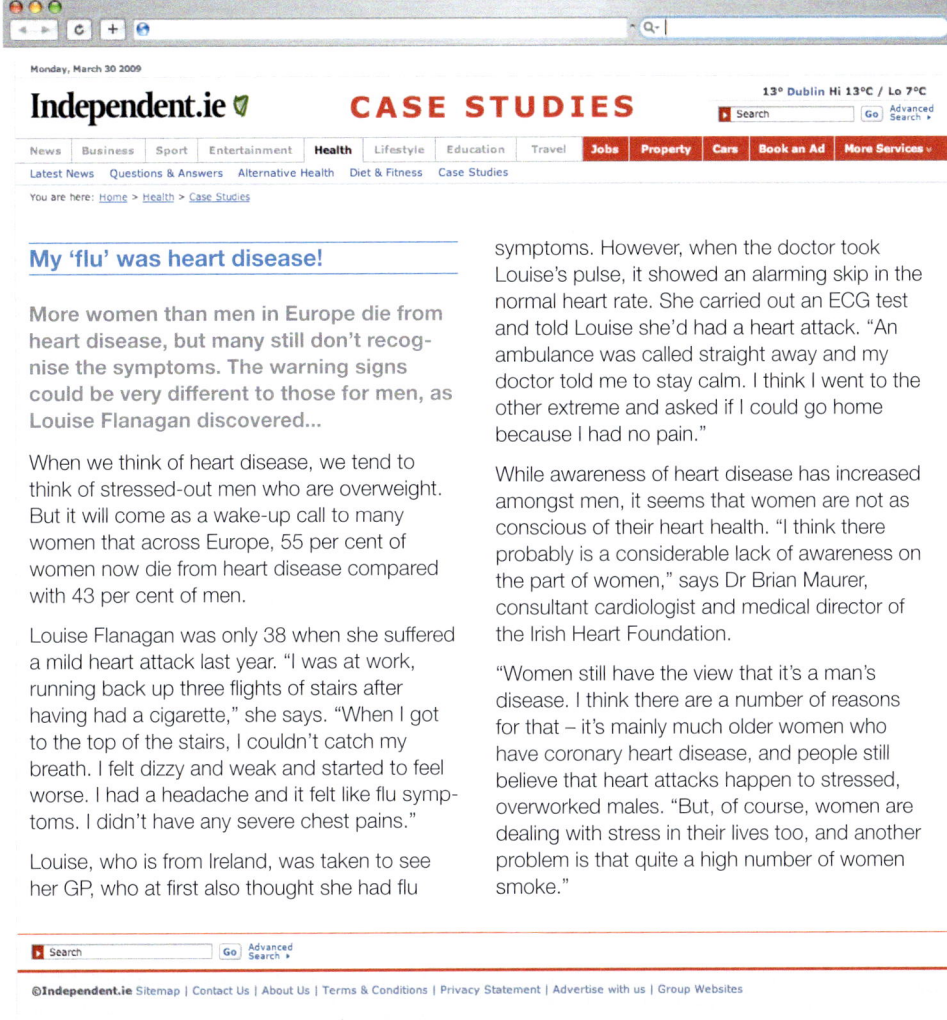

Monday, March 30 2009

Independent.ie

CASE STUDIES

13° Dublin Hi 13°C / Lo 7°C

News | Business | Sport | Entertainment | **Health** | Lifestyle | Education | Travel | **Jobs** | **Property** | **Cars** | **Book an Ad** | **More Services** v

Latest News   Questions & Answers   Alternative Health   Diet & Fitness   Case Studies

You are here: Home > Health > Case Studies

My 'flu' was heart disease!

More women than men in Europe die from heart disease, but many still don't recognise the symptoms. The warning signs could be very different to those for men, as Louise Flanagan discovered...

When we think of heart disease, we tend to think of stressed-out men who are overweight. But it will come as a wake-up call to many women that across Europe, 55 per cent of women now die from heart disease compared with 43 per cent of men.

Louise Flanagan was only 38 when she suffered a mild heart attack last year. "I was at work, running back up three flights of stairs after having had a cigarette," she says. "When I got to the top of the stairs, I couldn't catch my breath. I felt dizzy and weak and started to feel worse. I had a headache and it felt like flu symptoms. I didn't have any severe chest pains."

Louise, who is from Ireland, was taken to see her GP, who at first also thought she had flu symptoms. However, when the doctor took Louise's pulse, it showed an alarming skip in the normal heart rate. She carried out an ECG test and told Louise she'd had a heart attack. "An ambulance was called straight away and my doctor told me to stay calm. I think I went to the other extreme and asked if I could go home because I had no pain."

While awareness of heart disease has increased amongst men, it seems that women are not as conscious of their heart health. "I think there probably is a considerable lack of awareness on the part of women," says Dr Brian Maurer, consultant cardiologist and medical director of the Irish Heart Foundation.

"Women still have the view that it's a man's disease. I think there are a number of reasons for that – it's mainly much older women who have coronary heart disease, and people still believe that heart attacks happen to stressed, overworked males. "But, of course, women are dealing with stress in their lives too, and another problem is that quite a high number of women smoke."

©**Independent.ie** Sitemap | Contact Us | About Us | Terms & Conditions | Privacy Statement | Advertise with us | Group Websites

1 Who do people think is most likely to have a heart attack?
2 Why didn't Louise think she had heart disease?
3 What might have contributed to her heart disease?

2 In German

Use the information given in the text to design a leaflet for your German patients.

Treating a patient

1 Surgery equipment

Identify the medical supplies and equipment in the photos below.

examination gloves | hypodermic (syringe) | disinfectant | elastic bandage | thermometer | tourniquet | (a pair of) tweezers | (a pair of) scissors | gauze dressing | (cotton) swabs | scalpel | stethoscope | otoscope | blood-pressure cuff | surgical needle-holder | needle-thread combination

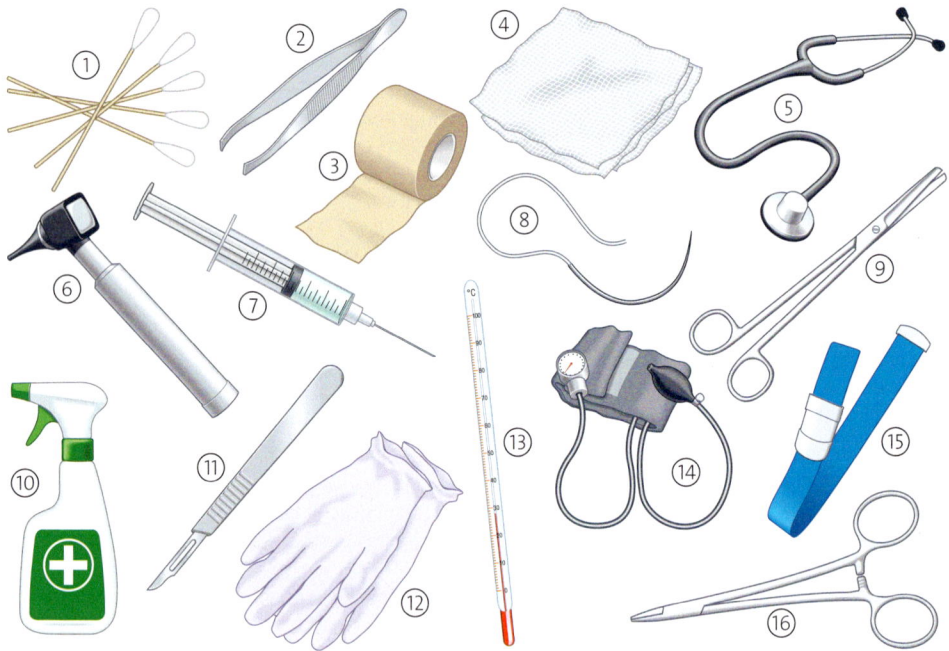

2 Working with words

Work with a partner. Use the words below to describe what each piece of equipment is used for.

take | give | clean | cut | stitch | dress | examine | extract | listen to | inject | protect | measure | ...

a wound | a dressing | a cut | blood | patients | the heartbeat | temperature | an injection | a sprain | ears | blood pressure | splinters | the skin | broken glass | hands | ...

A thermometer is used to take temperature.

Swabs are used for cleaning wounds.

You use a gauze dressing to dress a wound.

3 In the treatment room

Dr Grant and his nurse are treating a cut on a patient's arm. Describe what they are doing in each step and name the instruments they are using.

give local anaesthetic | take stitches out | examine wound |
tie off stitches | clean wound | dress wound | stitch wound

LANGUAGE Sequence words

First ... | Then ... | Next ... |
After that ... | Finally ...

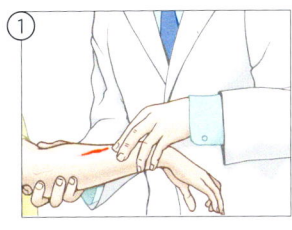

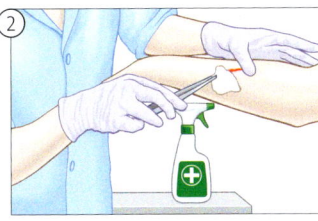

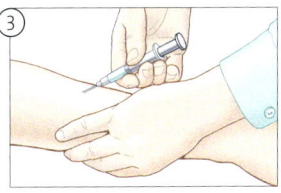

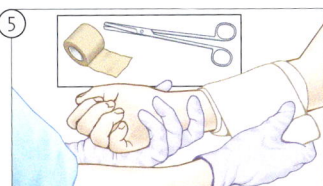

3

Ten days later

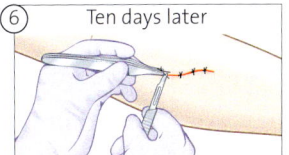

4 Stitching a wound

T13 Listen to the dialogue.

Then complete the following step-by-step description of the treatment.

1 First the doctor ...
2 Then he ...
3 The anaesthetic ...
4 While they waited, the nurse ...
5 She also ...
6 When the doctor returned, the nurse ...
7 The doctor ...
8 Then he ...
9 Finally, the nurse ...

cleaned
dressed
gave (2x)
got
stitched
talked to
tied off
took

a couple of minutes to take effect.
everything ready for the stitching procedure.
the cut/wound. (3x)
him a needle with thread and a needle holder.
Mr Carter a local anaesthetic.
the stitches.
Mr Carter and reassured him.

LANGUAGE Social skills

- Use their names when you greet patients.
  Good morning, Mr/Mrs ...
  How are you today?
- Reassure anxious patients.
  Don't worry.
  You'll hardly feel a thing.
  It won't take long.
- Some light 'small talk' can also help patients to relax.
  Have you lived here long?
  Do you know this area well?
- Make suitable sympathetic responses which show the patient that you are listening to them.
  That's wonderful/good/not so good/bad/terrible!

5 Practice

Complete the questions using the present continuous.

1 (get)   ... Caroline ... everything ready for the stitching procedure?
2 (treat) Which patient ... Dr Kingsley ... now?
3 (feel)   ... you still ... unwell, Mr Enderby?
4 (stop)   ... this medication still ... the pain, Mr Jones?
5 (wait) How many patients ... ... to see Dr Carey?

6 Taking blood

Mary Smith is one of Dr Müller's patients. She has got an appointment for an immunization. Before the doctor gives Mary the injection, she asks Kerstin to do a blood test.

Look at the illustrations and role play the dialogue between Mary and Kerstin.

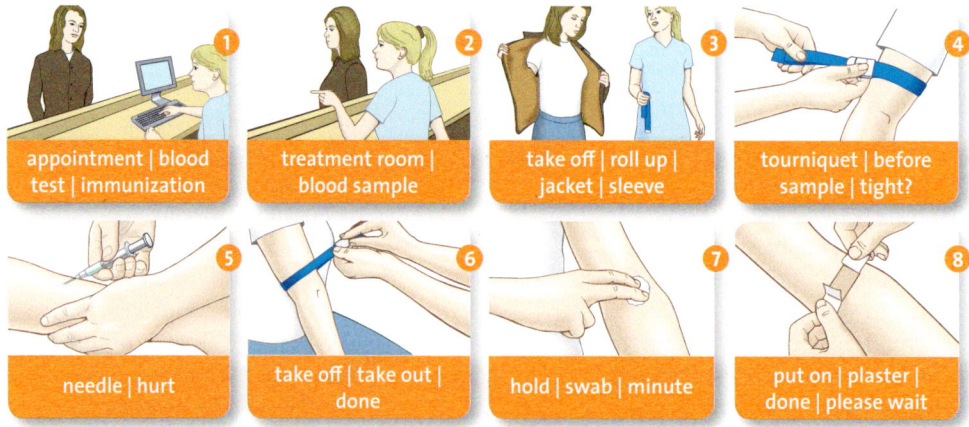

appointment | blood test | immunization	treatment room | blood sample	take off | roll up | jacket | sleeve	tourniquet | before sample | tight?
needle | hurt	take off | take out | done	hold | swab | minute	put on | plaster | done | please wait

T14 Now listen to the actual dialogue and check your results.

7 Taking blood pressure

A patient has an appointment for a check-up. Work with a partner to make a dialogue.

MFA	Patient/in

An der Rezeption

MFA	Patient/in
Begrüßen Sie den Patient/die Patientin.	
	Stellen Sie sich vor. Sagen Sie, dass Sie einen Termin für eine Vorsorgeunter-suchung haben.
Bestätigen Sie den Termin. Schicken Sie den Patienten/die Patientin in das Behandlungszimmer.	
	Fragen Sie, wo das Behandlungszimmer ist.
Erklären Sie den Weg. Sagen Sie, dass Sie gleich zum Blutdruckmessen kommen werden.	
	Stimmen Sie zu.

Im Behandlungszimmer

MFA	Patient/in
Bitten Sie den Patienten/die Patientin, die Jacke auszuziehen und den Ärmel hoch zu krempeln.	
	Fragen Sie, ob es so in Ordnung ist.
Erklären Sie, was Sie tun. Fragen Sie, ob es dem Patienten/der Patientin gut geht.	
	Bestätigen Sie, dass alles bestens ist.
Entfernen Sie die Blutdruckmanschette. Teilen Sie dem Patienten/der Patientin den Blutdruckwert mit: 150/90 mm Hg.	
	Bitten Sie die MFA um Erklärung, ob der Wert in Ordnung ist.
Erklären Sie, dass der Wert zu hoch ist und Sie den Arzt/die Ärztin informieren werden.	
	Sagen Sie, dass Ihr Blutdruck normaler-weise niedrig ist.
Beruhigen Sie den Patienten /die Patientin.	
	Danken Sie der MFA/dem MFA.

8 Parts of the body

Match these parts of the body with the numbers in the illustrations.

ankle | appendix | back | buttocks | chest | chin | shin | elbow |
hip | jaw | kidneys | knee | liver | lungs | neck | shoulder |
stomach | thigh | throat | wrist | knuckle | spleen

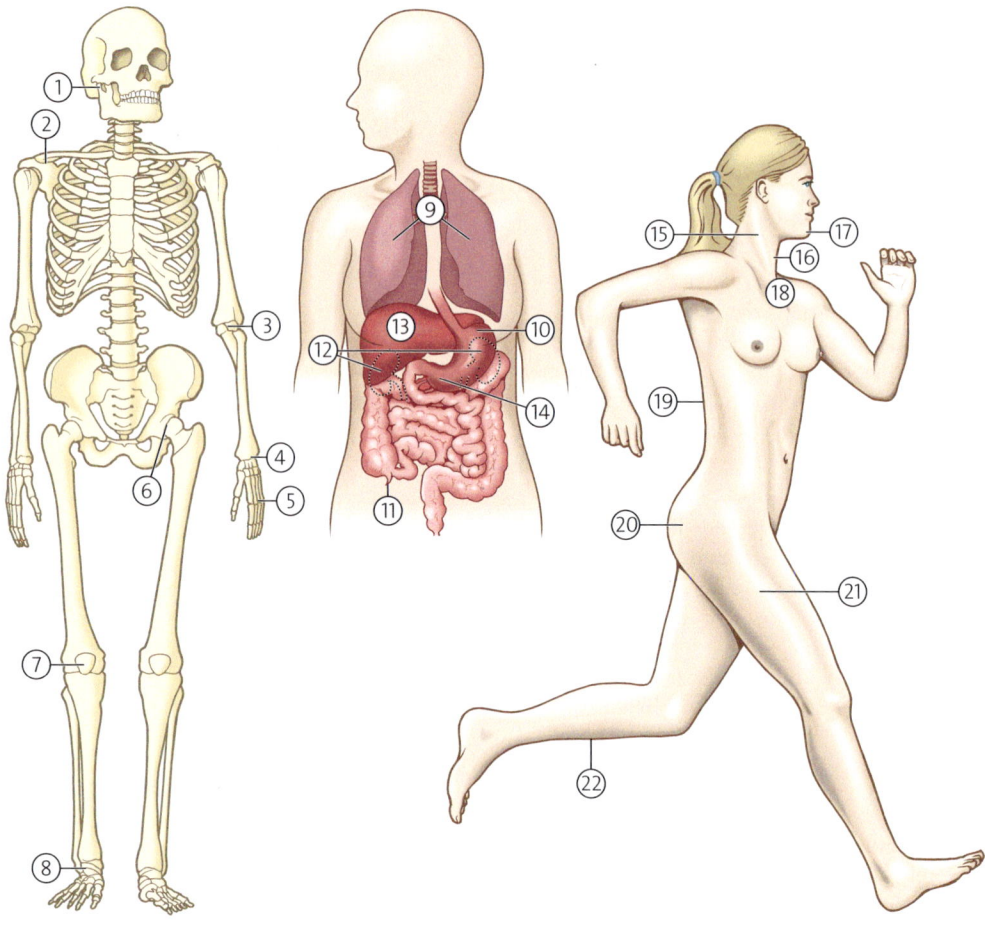

Copy this table into your exercise book and complete it.

Joints	Organs	Other body parts

9 Practice

Work with a partner. One student thinks of an organ, a joint or a part of the body
and the other guesses what it is by asking questions.

Extra material

1 True or false?

Read the information in this text about the use of video conferencing in the UK. Are the statements below true or false? Correct the false statements.

The future of remote medical consultations

Connecting doctors with patients by video is not new – but is now the time for it finally to take off?

Aberdeen Royal Infirmary in Scotland is conducting an experiment in telemedicine – diagnosing and treating medical conditions by video conferencing. The trial is to check whether teleconsultations are as good as face-to-face ones.

The technology is a video conferencing system which presents a life-size high-definition image of the patient as if they were sitting just across the table. The patient's booth includes medical devices – such as a stethoscope, blood-pressure cuff and thermometer – to send important information to the doctor. The whole setup works on a standard broadband network and the experience is very close to life. "It was just like a normal consultation", says a patient.

Patients who volunteer for teleconsultations also have face-to-face examinations. The next stage will be to move the patient booth to a "remote safe site",

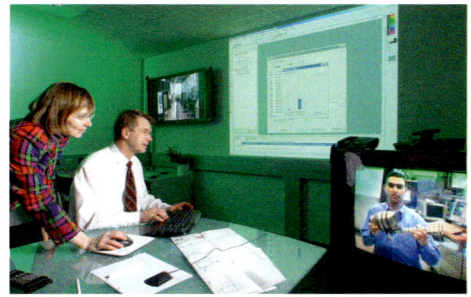

probably a community hospital, where hands-on medical help is available. If that works, the booth could go almost anywhere – maybe even in a hotel or a police station.

Even if the trials succeed, creating a full service may be difficult. Setting up a sponsored pilot trial is one thing, running an ongoing service across the whole NHS is quite another. The lesson of 50 years of telemedicine is that, even if the technology can work, it is only one part of a much larger jigsaw.

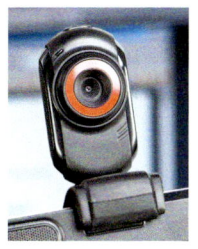

1. The trials are taking place in three UK hospitals.
2. The trial is to see how good the face-to-face consultations are.
3. There is medical equipment in the patient booth.
4. The system uses special network technology.
5. Patients in the trial also have face-to-face consultations.
6. The booths will only be used in hospitals.
7. If the trial is successful, booths will be used all over the UK.

2 Activity

Your boss has asked you to give him a summary of the article. Make notes in your exercise book under these headings.

what is happening | where | what is the system | how does it work | what happens next

At a pharmacy

1 Filling a prescription

T 15

Julie Peters goes to a pharmacy in Hamburg to get a prescription filled for a hepatitis A injection. Katrin Scholl works there as a pharmacist.

Listen to the dialogue on the CD and then complete the summary below. Write the missing words in your exercise book.

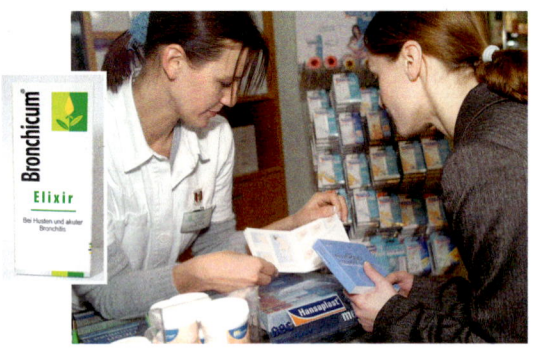

Julie has a ...[1] from her doctor. She asks the ...[2] to give her something for a ...[3]. She's got a ...[4] cough. Katrin asks Julie if she has any other ...[5]. Julie tells her that she also has a bit of a ...[6]. Katrin warns her that if she has the ...[7], her doctor won't be able to give her the ...[8] against ...[9]. Katrin gives Julie some over-the-counter cough mixture for her ...[10] and some ...[11] tablets for her headache.

Julie can't read the ...[12] on the packet. Katrin tells her that she can take a tablet three or four ...[13] a day, but not more than ...[14] in one day. She can take one or two ...[15] of the cough ...[16] every ...[17] hours.

T 15

Check your answers by listening to the dialogue on the CD again.

2 Products at a pharmacy

You can buy all the products in the list below at a pharmacy.

Work with a partner:

1 What are the German names for these products?

2 Which of the products below can you buy over the counter in a German pharmacy and which are available only on prescription?

antibiotics | paracetamol | suntan lotion | contraceptive pills | cosmetics | cough medicine | hepatitis vaccine | insulin | painkillers | sleeping tablets | laxative | anti-depressants | cough sweets | antihistamine

'Antibiotics' are called 'Antibiotika' in German.

You	can buy ...	over the counter.
	can't buy ...	at a supermarket.
	need	a doctor's prescription for ... .
Cosmetics	can be bought	without a doctor's prescription.
Insulin	can't be bought	over the counter.
...	can only be bought	with a doctor's prescription.

1 The pharmacist **fills** the customer's prescription.
2 The customer's prescription **is filled** by the pharmacist.
3 You **must take** a red capsule after every meal.
4 A red capsule **must be taken** after every meal.
5 **Are** effervescent tablets **sold** over the counter in British pharmacies?
6 The assistant **doesn't accept** the customer's American credit card.
7 The customer's American credit card **isn't accepted**.

- Aktive Sätze (1, 3, 6) sagen, wer die Handlung (nicht) ausgeführt hat.
- Die Passivformen (2, 4, 7) betonen dagegen die Handlung – die Person, die sie ausführt, ist nicht so wichtig und kann sogar weggelassen werden.
- Die *simple present*-Passivform von Vollverben ist *is/are* + Partizip Perfekt (2, 5).
- Die Negation im Passiv wird mit *isn't/aren't* + Partizip Perfekt gebildet (7).
- Fragen im Passiv fangen mit dem Hilfsverb *Is/Are ...?* an (5).

3 Practice

 First look at the active sentences. Then complete the passive sentences.

1 Does the nurse order supplies for the practice?
... supplies for the practice ordered by the nurse?
2 Doctor Scott gives the patient an injection.
The patient ... given an injection.
3 The nurse asks Mrs Shipton for a urine sample.
Mrs Shipton ... ... for a urine sample.
4 A nurse takes Mr Daley to a treatment room.
Mr Daley ... ... to a treatment room.
5 Does your health insurance cover physiotherapy?
... physiotherapy ... by your health insurance?
6 The doctor always warns patients about the side effects of their medication.
The patients ... always ... about the side effects of their medication.

4 What are they?

Can you identify the six illustrations below?

capsule | drops | throat pastilles | sugared pill | tablet | effervescent tablet

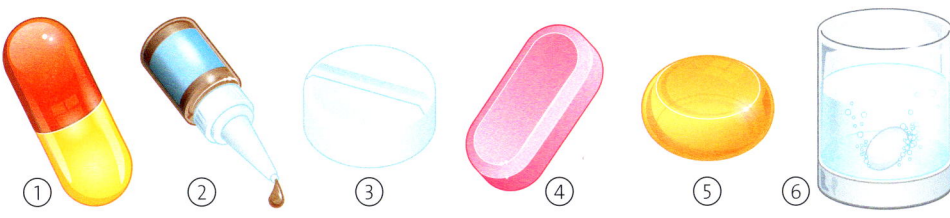

5 Dosage instructions

Give an English-speaking patient the dosage instructions and any other important information from the products below. Leave out any information you don't think is so important. The words and phrases in the box below can help you.

1 **Dosierungsanleitung, Art und Dauer der Anwendung**
Soweit nichts anders verordnet, 3–5-mal täglich 20–30 Tropfen (½ Teelöffel) mit etwas Flüssigkeit oder auf Zucker vor den Mahlzeiten einnehmen. Die Anwendung erfolgt bis zur Beendigung der Beschwerden.

2 Eine Tablette einmal täglich während der Mahlzeit einnehmen. Nicht auf nüchternen Magen einnehmen, da Magenbeschwerden und Übelkeit auftreten können.

3 3–4-mal täglich 1 Kapsel eine halbe Stunde vor dem Essen mit reichlich kalter Flüssigkeit einnehmen. Zur Erleichterung der Nachtruhe kann die letzte Dosis vor dem Schlafengehen eingenommen werden.

4 **Nebenwirkungen**
Im seltenen Fällen Magenbeschwerden und Übelkeit.

5 Erwachsene und Jugendliche ab 14 Jahren nehmen 2–3-mal täglich 1 Brausetablette ein. Kinder von 2–5 Jahren nehmen 3-mal täglich ½ Brausetablette oder 2-mal täglich 1 Brausetablette ein. Die Brausetabletten werden nach den Mahlzeiten in ½ Glas Wasser aufgelöst und die Lösung getrunken. Bei akuten Erkrankungen werden die Brausetabletten im Allgemeinen über 5–7 Tage eingenommen. Die Dauer der Behandlung richtet sich nach Art und Schwere der Erkrankung und sollte vom behandelnden Arzt bestimmt werden.

LANGUAGE **Taking medicine**

Unless otherwise prescribed …
Take with/before/after/meals.
Take once or twice a day.
Take a pill regularly every three hours.

This capsule should be taken with some/ lots of fluid/water.

Do not take on an empty stomach/with other medication.

Dissolve in water. / Allow to dissolve in the mouth.
Swallow the tablet with water.

Side effects: in a minority of cases this medicine may cause …
drowsiness/nausea/stomach complaints/ blurred vision/…

Be careful!
In English you take something *for* a headache or a back pain – **not** *against*.

6 Ordering supplies

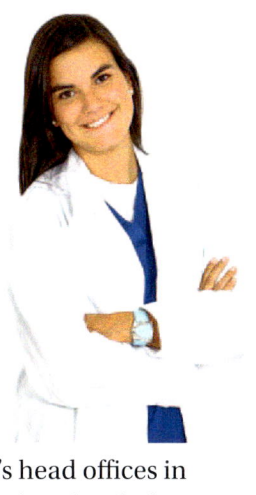

Sarila Yildiz works as a medical assistant in Dr Fischer's practice. One of her jobs is ordering supplies from an international pharmaceutical supply company. Unfortunately, there are sometimes mistakes with orders.

 T 16 Listen to Sarila talking to an assistant at the supply company's head offices in Rotterdam. Compare what she ordered with the delivery note and find out what is wrong with the shipment.

There should be ... and not ...

Sarila ordered ... and not ...

Verhoeven Pharmaceutical Supplies	
Delivery Note 25607/A23	
No.	Item
20	0,5 litre bottles of saline infusion
20	infusion pumps
150	doses of tetanus vaccine
4	boxes of gauze bandages
2	boxes of examination gloves
50	disposable syringes
1	1 litre bottle of general disinfectant
3	50 g tins of antiseptic ointment

Write the corrected delivery note in an exercise book.

7 Serving a customer

Work with a partner to make a dialogue.

Apotheker/in	Kunde/Kundin
Begrüßen Sie den Kunden/die Kundin.	Fragen Sie nach einem Mittel gegen Kopfschmerzen.
Fragen Sie nach den Symptomen.	Sagen Sie, dass es Ihnen im Stirnbereich weh tut und Sie außerdem Halsschmerzen haben.
Empfehlen Sie einige Produkte, z. B. Brausetabletten, Tropfen, Dragees, Lutschtabletten.	Fragen Sie nach der Dosierung, Art und Dauer der Anwendungen.
Beantworten Sie die Fragen.	Fragen Sie nach Nebenwirkungen.
Beantworten Sie die Frage.	Fragen Sie nach den Kosten.
Sagen Sie den Preis. Fragen Sie nach weiteren Wünschen.	Verneinen Sie und bezahlen Sie die Medikamente.
Bedanken Sie sich und verabschieden Sie sich von dem Kunden/der Kundin.	Danken Sie für die Hilfe und verabschieden Sie sich.

8 Saying where things are

Look at the street map below. Where are the following places?

bank | pharmacy | hospital | cinema | optician | shopping centre | bus station

next to | opposite | between | on the corner of ... and ... | near to | at the end of

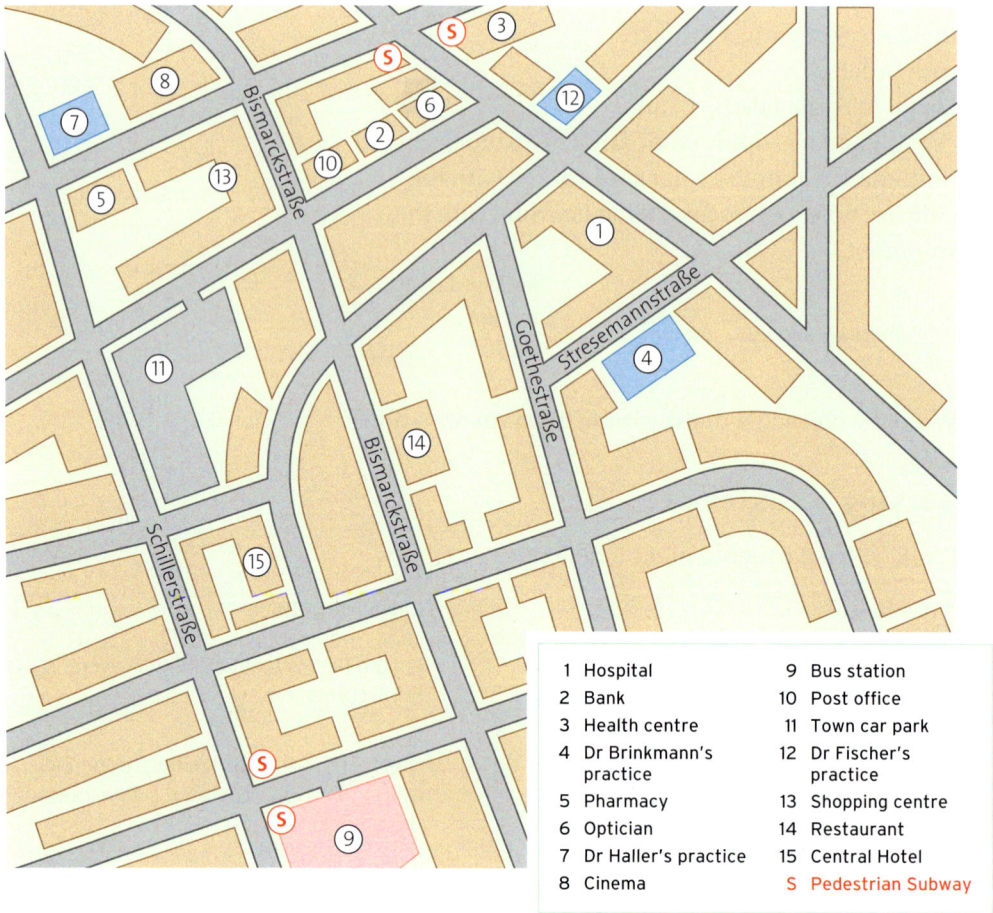

1	Hospital	9	Bus station
2	Bank	10	Post office
3	Health centre	11	Town car park
4	Dr Brinkmann's practice	12	Dr Fischer's practice
5	Pharmacy	13	Shopping centre
6	Optician	14	Restaurant
7	Dr Haller's practice	15	Central Hotel
8	Cinema	S	Pedestrian Subway

9 Giving directions

T 17 Listen to a medical receptionist giving directions to a patient. Draw a sketch of the instructions she gives him. Find the starting point and the finishing point on the map.

LANGUAGE Directions

Turn left/right (at the ...)
first/second/third/fourth crossroads.
The ... is on your left/right.

Walk along ... until you reach (the) ...
You'll see a/an ...
There's a/an ...

---

10 Another medical practice

Read the dialogue and find this practice on the map on page 36.
Then, in your exercise book complete the dialogue with the directions.

Patient Can you tell me how to get to the bus station from here, please?

Nurse Yes, certainly. Do you want to walk or take the bus?

Patient I'd prefer to walk, if it isn't too far.

Nurse It'll take you about twenty minutes on foot.

Patient That's fine. I've got plenty of time.

Nurse OK. When you leave here, cross the road to the pharmacy on the corner.

Patient Oh, yes. I saw it when I came in.

Nurse OK. So then you …

T18 Now listen to the complete dialogue and check your directions.

Role play the dialogue with a partner.

11 Arranging a meeting

Work with a partner. Choose a place on the map on page 36 and then call your
partner with your mobile phone. Tell him/her where you are. Ask where he/she is
and then tell him/her how to reach you.

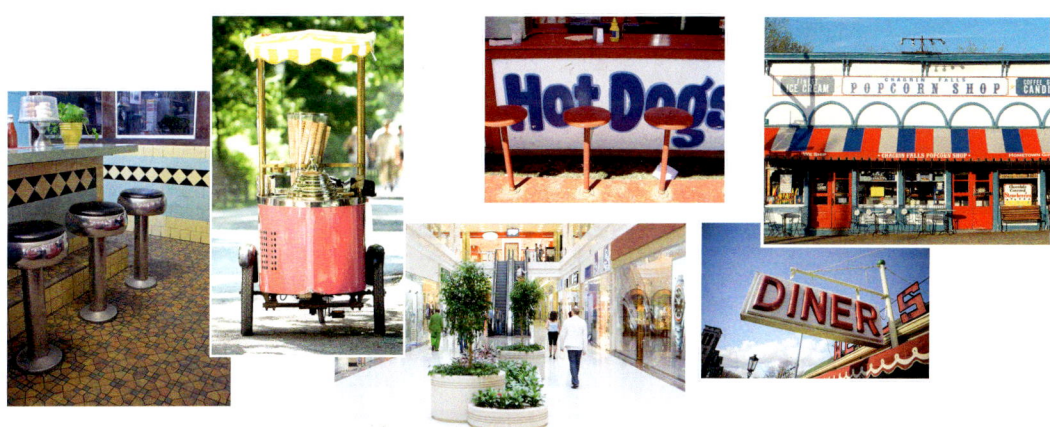

LANGUAGE Small talk	
Would you like to join me?	The bargains/food/people/… here are
I'm standing/sitting/in/in front of/a/an …	fantastic/fun/delicious/cheap/unusual/…
I've found a really interesting …	It's opposite/next to/near the …
Do you fancy meeting me here for a …?	diner/hot dog cart/candy shop/…
I thought it would be nice to meet here	It's such a wonderful/interesting/… place.
because …	The weather is so warm/sunny/pleasant/…

1 Sexually Transmitted Diseases

Read the information about the rise of HIV infections in the UK and then say what the following numbers refer to.

a quarter | 40,000 | 1,000 | 376,508 | 21,698 | 16%

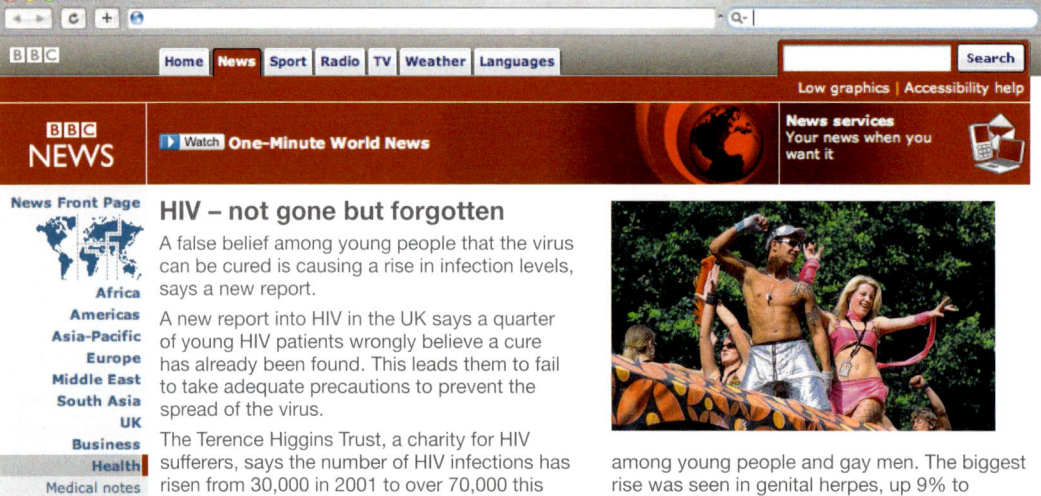

BBC | Home | News | Sport | Radio | TV | Weather | Languages

Search

Low graphics | Accessibility help

BBC NEWS

▶ Watch **One-Minute World News**

News services
Your news when you want it

News Front Page

Africa
Americas
Asia-Pacific
Europe
Middle East
South Asia
UK
Business
Health
Medical notes
Science & Environment
Technology
Entertainment
Also in the news

HIV – not gone but forgotten

A false belief among young people that the virus can be cured is causing a rise in infection levels, says a new report.

A new report into HIV in the UK says a quarter of young HIV patients wrongly believe a cure has already been found. This leads them to fail to take adequate precautions to prevent the spread of the virus.

The Terence Higgins Trust, a charity for HIV sufferers, says the number of HIV infections has risen from 30,000 in 2001 to over 70,000 this year. Research by the charity in July suggested there was still widespread ignorance about HIV, especially amongst young people. A poll of 1,000 people found that more than 20% of people aged 18–24 mistakenly thought there was a cure for HIV.

The rise in HIV is part of a wider trend. A Health Protection Agency (HPA) report found diagnoses of new sexually transmitted diseases (STDs) rose by 2% to 376,508 in 2006, largely among young people and gay men. The biggest rise was seen in genital herpes, up 9% to 21,698. Among young girls aged 16–19, the rise was 16%. Sexual infection diagnoses have risen almost continually since the 1990s, with the highest increases in recent years in the 16–24 age group.

The HPA said part of the rise was due to more people having tests. Dr Gwen Taylor, head of the HPA, also said higher STD rates were found in young people because they were more sexually active.

© BBC MMIX | Most Popular Now | 29,800 pages were read in the last minute. | Back to top ^^

Help | Privacy and cookies policy | News sources | About the BBC | Contact us |

2 Content

Answer the following questions about the text.

1 Why is the number of HIV infections rising in the UK?
2 Who made this information public?
3 What is the fastest growing sexually transmitted infection?
4 Which group has experienced the largest rise in diagnoses for genital herpes?
5 Why is the overall rate of diagnoses of sexually transmitted infections growing?

3 Problem words

Complete the sentences by choosing the correct words from the box.

1. The doctor gave me ... for a painkiller.
2. A patient phoned the health centre to make ...
3. Could you ... down on the examination couch, please?
4. I need some ... details.
5. A patient was sick and looked very ...
6. The nurse put a ... on the wound.
7. Could you ... your arm, please?
8. I forgot to ask for a ... when I bought the vaccine.
9. I didn't get the number because the patient phoned from a ...
10. You need to take the pills ... a day.

> (a/an ...) appointment | binding |
> date | dressing | handy | lay | lie |
> mobile | personal | personnel |
> prescription | receipt | raise |
> recipe | rise | two times | twice |
> unhappy | unlucky

4 The dangers of HIV

How do you protect yourself and others from HIV:

a) in your private life and
b) in your practice?

Prepare a presentation.

> www.avert.org/aids-help-uk.htm
> www.aidshelpline.org.za/
> www.muktaahivhelpline.org/
> www.aids-info.ch

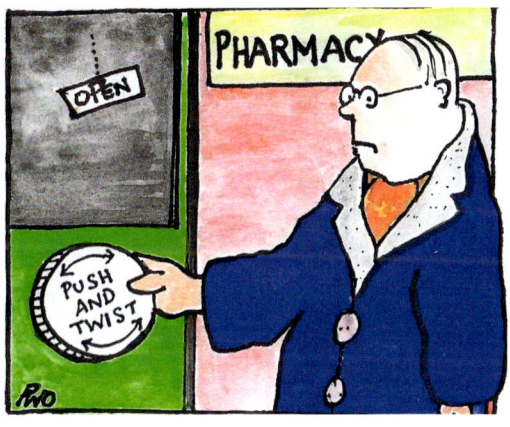

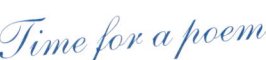

Time for a poem

Give me a doctor partridge-plump,
Short in the leg and broad in the rump,
An endomorph with gentle hands
Who'll never make absurd demands
That I abandon all my vices
Nor pull a long face in a crisis,
But with a twinkle in his eye
will tell me that I have to die.

W. H. AUDEN 1907–73

partridge	Rebhuhn
plump	dicklich
endomorph	Pykniker (rund- licher Körpertyp)
demands	Forderungen
abandon	aufgeben
vices	Laster
twinkle	Glitzern

6 Communication

1 Different people have different needs

T19 These people are in the waiting room of your practice. Listen and find out who they are and why they are there.

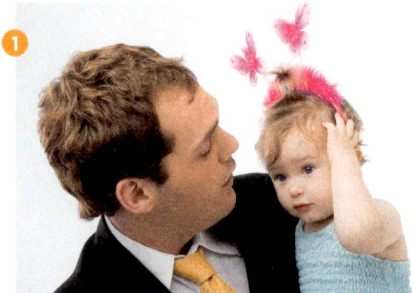

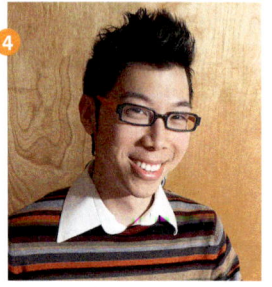

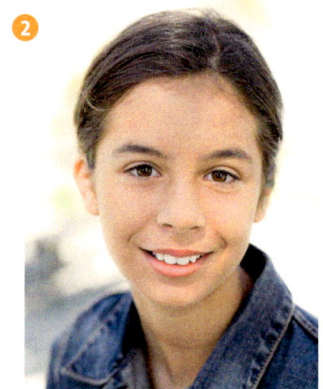

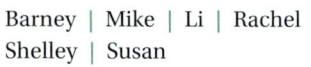

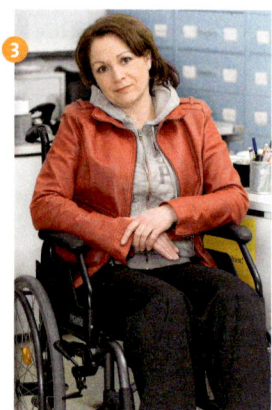

Barney | Mike | Li | Rachel | Shelley | Susan

back pain | blood and urine samples | pelvic examination | prescription medication | smallpox vaccination | tetanus injection

Photo 1 shows …

What special needs do you think these patients might have? Think about health problems, language difficulties, cultural differences, physical and mental needs. Make suggestions about how you could help them.

I notice that … needs/has got a	hearing aid. wheelchair. pushchair. Chinese name. …

He/She	is looks seems must be …	disabled. partially deaf. anxious. nervous. …

I	can could	give … bring … help … with help … to take … to …	a toy. a magazine. getting out of … undress. the toilet. an explanation. …

40 Unit 6

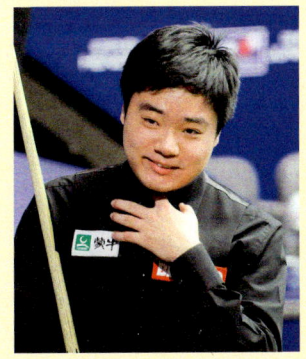

In traditional Chinese names the family name comes first. So 'Gao Chang' is 'Mr Gao' and **not** 'Mr Chang'. However, Chinese emigrants to western countries as well as many Chinese business-men and people from Hongkong and Singapore often use a 'Western' first name and put their family name last, e.g. Edward Gao, Betty Wan, etc.

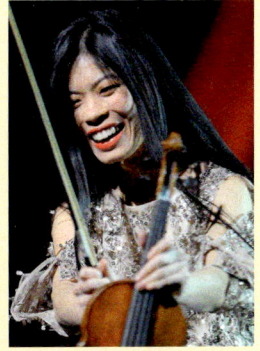

Ding Junhui, snooker champion

Vanessa Mae, violinist

2 What makes us anxious?

Everyone feels anxious sometimes. How anxious do the following situations make you feel? Rate them on a scale of 1 to 5 (1 = relaxed, 2 = nervous, 3 = tense, 4 = worried, 5 = very anxious).

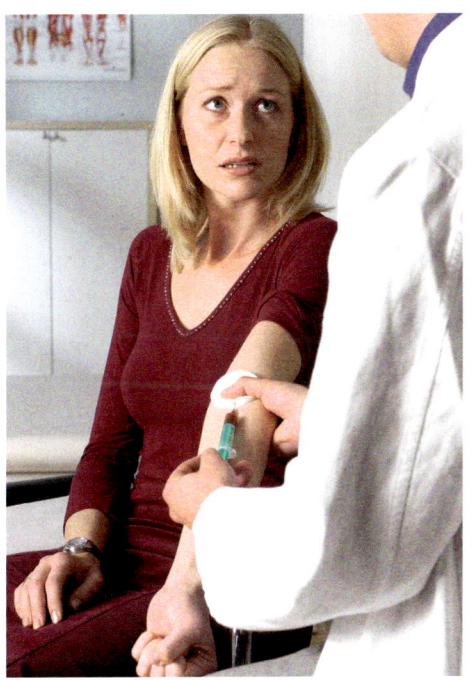

a) speaking English
b) having dental treatment
c) taking an English exam
d) travelling by plane
e) a job interview
f) having an injection

Expressing anxiety

I'm afraid of / scared of / anxious about …
… makes me nervous / feel uncomfortable.
I worry about …

3 Patient anxiety

Read the text on the next page and match the paragraphs with the headings below.

a) Fear of physical pain
b) No news is good news
c) Anxiety about illness and death
d) Poor communication skills
e) Fear of infection

Are you anxious in the doctor's office?

Millions of Americans hate visiting the doctor. They are often afraid of visiting the doctor's office or a hospital because such places have a certain smell and atmosphere to them. They can smell of medicine and that can be scary for some people.

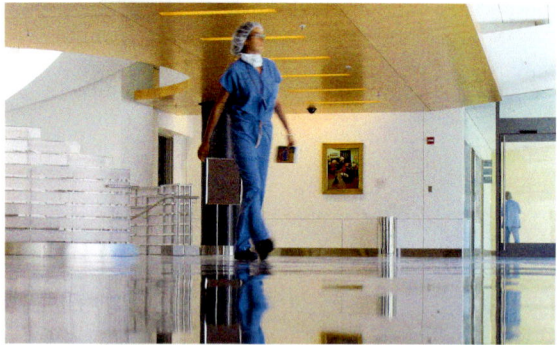

1 ...

Another common cause of anxiety is the fact that a doctor's office and a hospital are where people are sick and suffering from diseases such as cancer and other life-threatening conditions. Some people are uncomfortable when around others who are seriously ill.

2 ...

Many people are scared of doctors themselves. Doctors often have a certain kind of 'coldness' to them. They are trained not to be emotional and that can scare patients. When doctors are cold and don't seem friendly, patients can feel as if they are just another number on a sheet of paper.

3 ...

A lot of people are scared of the doctor because they associate the doctor with painful things, such as injections and needles. People often don't understand what their treatment involves and so feel helpless because they have no control over what is going to happen.

4 ...

Also, doctors can find out very scary things about us. We often go to see our doctor with symptoms but no idea about the cause. Sometimes, a doctor may give us bad news and we are afraid that there is something very seriously wrong with us. Many people would rather not hear the truth.

5 ...

Many people also think going to the doctor or visiting a hospital is a health risk. They think places full of sick people are also full of germs and they are worried about catching something and becoming sicker than when they went in.

4 True or false?

Read the text again and say whether the following statements are true or false. Correct the false statements in an exercise book.

1 Not many Americans worry about going to the doctor's office.
2 A cool clinical atmosphere makes patients feel comfortable.
3 A lot of people don't like being around other sick people.
4 Doctors are trained to be cold and unfriendly.
5 Fear of pain is another common reason for being nervous.
6 Patients don't want the doctor to explain the treatment to them.
7 When people don't know what's wrong with them, they fear the worst.
8 Some patients think they will get germs from visiting the practice.

5 Adjectives and nouns

Complete the table with the correct form of the words from the text.

	adjective	noun
1	anxious	...
2	...	discomfort
3	...	illness
4	...	emotion
5	...	pain
6	...	helplessness
7	afraid	...
8	...	worry
9	smelly	...
10	...	scare
11	risky	...

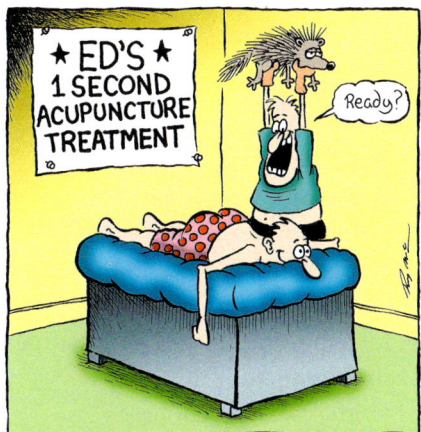

6 Working with words

Now complete the sentences with the correct form of the words.

1 Many patients would like their doctor to show more ... .
2 I was ... about my treatment but my doctor explained it very carefully.
3 Some patients feel ... because they have no control over what is happening.
4 With training, giving injections shouldn't be ... for patients.
5 Many people feel ... when faced with people who are seriously ill.
6 Some people are ... of the clinical atmosphere of a surgery.
7 Many adults suffer from ... when going to the doctor.
8 Some people think they can catch a serious ... at the doctor's.
9 'Frank N. Stein' is a very ... name for a doctor!
10 There is an element of ... in any surgical operation.
11 Women usually have a better sense of ... than men.

7 Scary medical instruments

Match the names with the instruments below.

bronchoscope | artery forceps | injection needle/syringe | speculum

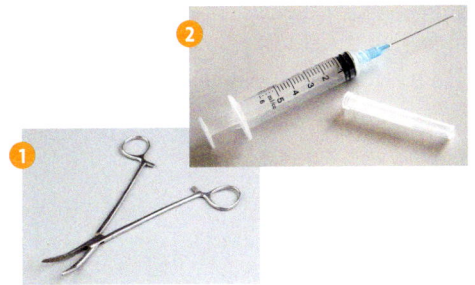

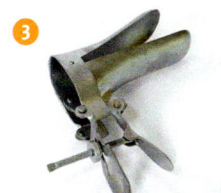

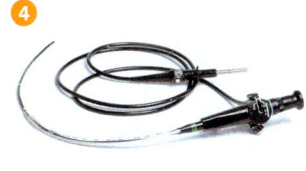

8 How to deal with anxiety

Look at the list of ways of dealing with patient anxiety.
What, in your opinion, is the most useful advice?
Rank the examples from 1 = 'the most useful' to 10 = 'the least useful'.

a) relaxing music
b) general anaesthetic
c) listening to the patient
d) watching TV during treatment
e) explaining the treatment fully
f) using modern instruments
g) relaxing foot spa
h) relaxing atmosphere in the surgery
i) massaging the patient
j) aromatherapy candles

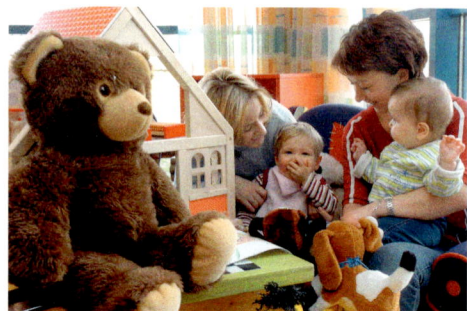

A waiting room with a children's play corner

9 Dealing with anxious patients

T 20 ⊙ Listen to Dr Graham talk about patient anxiety and how doctors deal with it nowadays. Match the improvements to how things were 30 years ago.

30 years ago	today
1 injections were painful	a) doctors listen to patients more
2 doctors had less time for patients	b) smaller needles
3 doctors didn't explain things to patients	c) surgeries have TVs and music
4 big scary instruments	d) doctors should take more time to explain treatments
5 not a relaxed atmosphere	e) smaller and less invasive instruments

Now write sentences with your answers.

Start like this
1 In the past injections and taking blood were painful but now needles are smaller and cause less pain.
2 Thirty years ago, doctors couldn't spend as much time talking to their patients.

10 Over to you

T 20 ⊙ What are patients worried about now when they visit the doctor?
Listen to Dr Graham again and make notes. Then add your own ideas.

Nervous anxious patients need ...	We could offer ...
lots of | information	We should have ...
reassurance	... would be a good idea.
...	... might help.

1 Doctors **should** always explain the risks and the benefits of each treatment.
2 The patients **have (got) to** trust you or they **shouldn't** start the treatment.
3 Some doctors think great anaesthetics mean they **don't have to** talk to their patients!
4 With today's anaesthetics, patients really **needn't** feel any pain at all.
5 Doctors **mustn't** forget to listen to their patients.

- ***Should*** drückt einen Ratschlag oder eine Empfehlung aus (1).
- ***Must*** und ***have (got) to*** drücken eine Notwendigkeit bzw. Verpflichtung aus (2).
  Die Verneinung von ***must/have to*** ist ***don't have to*** (3) bzw. ***needn't*** (4).
- Vorsicht: ***mustn't*** drückt ein Verbot aus (5) und bedeutet 'nicht dürfen'.

11 Practice

Choose the correct verb to complete the sentences.

1 With modern anaesthetics patients *needn't/mustn't* feel any pain.
2 Some doctors think they *don't have to/mustn't* listen to their patients.
3 Doctors *shouldn't/needn't* leave instruments lying around the surgery.
4 Patients *don't have to/must* go on with treatment if they feel nervous.
5 The sterilization centre *mustn't/needn't* be in the same room as the surgery.
6 Patients *don't have to/shouldn't* have a reason for feeling anxious.
7 A doctor *needn't/shouldn't* look rushed or too busy.
8 People who are nervous about treatment *needn't/must* tell their doctor.

12 Situations

Work with a partner. Think of examples for the following things.

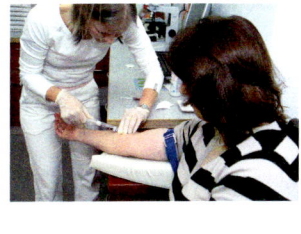

Something you …
1 … shouldn't do at work.
2 … don't have to do at home (but your partner does).
3 … must do every day at work (but your partner doesn't).
4 … have to do this weekend.

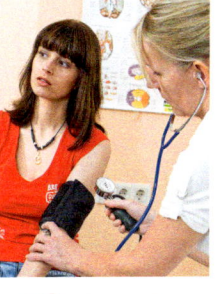

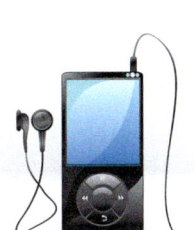

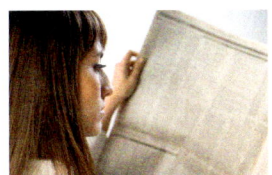

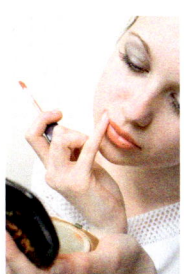

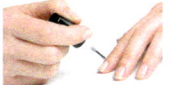

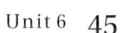

13 The pelvic exam

Work with a partner. Discuss the following questions in German.

1 Why is it a good idea for young women to have a pelvic exam regularly?
2 When should a young woman go to the doctor for her first pelvic exam?
3 How often should she then have regular pelvic exams?

14 A first pelvic exam

T 21 Susan Farrows, 16, has arrived at the doctor's for her first pelvic exam. Meike, the medical assistant at reception, talks to her. Listen and take notes on what happens during the exam.

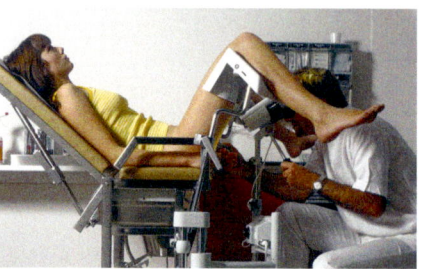

LANGUAGE Reassuring patients
There's nothing to worry about.
Don't worry, it's just a …
It's just a …, it won't hurt.
It's a very routine test / procedure / operation.
It's perfectly normal.

15 A young patient

Work with a partner. A fifteen-year-old Australian girl comes to your surgery for an HPV* exam and vaccination. Make up a dialogue between her and the medical assistant.

Medical assistant	Girl
Greet the girl and ask for name and appointment time.	
	Greet receptionist and give your name and the time of your appointment.
Ask if it is her first visit to the surgery.	
	Say no, you have been before for a pelvic exam.
Ask if the appointment is for another check up.	
	No, this time it is for an HPV* exam and a vaccination.
Ask if she is feeling anxious.	
	No, you aren't anxious, but you are a bit nervous.
Reassure her by explaining the procedure.	

* HPV = human papilloma virus

Extra material

1 The patient-carer relationship

You are going to hear Joyce Reynolds give a presentation to people training to work in health and social care about the relationship between patients and carers.

Before listening, work with a partner to make a list of things that can go wrong in a patient-carer relationship. How do you think these problems can be avoided?

Now listen to the talk and put these headings into the correct order.

be honest | let clients do things for themselves | look after yourself | be patient and calm | take time to listen

2 Working with words

Listen again and match the verbs (1–6) with the nouns and phrases (a–f).

1 show
2 get
3 keep
4 don't reduce
5 tell
6 take

a) their self-respect
b) the truth
c) warmth
d) care of yourself
e) calm
f) angry

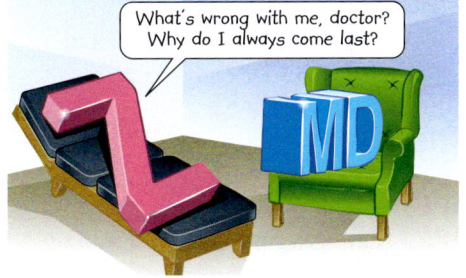

What's wrong with me, doctor? Why do I always come last?

3 Mediation

Give a presentation to the class about the relationship between a medical assistant and patients at the practice. What kind of communication problems can occur and how can you avoid or solve them?

These websites can help you:

www.yahoo.co.uk/society_and_culture/disabilities — Here you can find links to other websites about various disabilities.

www.rnib.org.uk — The Royal National Institute for the Blind is the UK's largest support organization for the blind.

www.housingcare.org — Information, advice and useful links about rest homes for the elderly.

www.elderconnect.com — A database of US care providers for the elderly.

www.retirement-living.com — General information about retirement in the USA: health issues, living at home, care services.

1 Healthy eating quiz

Work with a partner. Look at the questions and decide which is the correct answer.

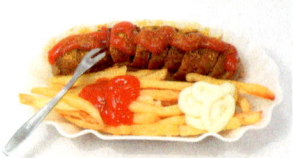

Question 1

How often should you eat fish, according to experts?

- A: once a week
- B: twice a week
- C: every day

Question 2

What contains the most vitamin C?

- A: plums
- B: oranges
- C: kiwis

Question 3

How much water do experts reckon people should drink every day?

- A: 1 litre
- B: 2 litres
- C: 3 litres

Question 4

How much calcium do our bodies need to be healthy?

- A: 250 mg per day
- B: 500 mg per day
- C: 1000 mg per day

Question 5

What percentage of our daily calorie intake (energy) should come from carbohydrates?

- A: more than 50 per cent
- B: more than 80 per cent
- C: 100 per cent

LANGUAGE Agreeing and disagreeing

How do you feel about ...?
I think that's right/wrong. What about you?
Do you agree?
I agree (with you).
I'm sorry, I don't agree./ I disagree.
I think ...

2 A healthy diet

Match the food items below to the six food groups in the healthy diet chart. Which food items can't be matched to the chart? Then add three items to each group. Use a dictionary to help you.

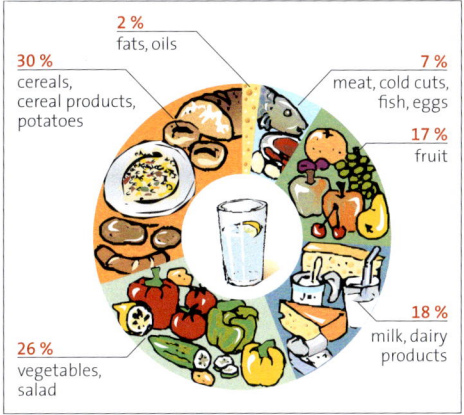

spaghetti | bananas | salt | cream |
sugar | wine | cornflakes | chocolate |
biscuits | bread rolls | orange juice |
beer | salmon | chicken | broccoli |
cola | sausage | onions | maple syrup

Complete this sentence:
Food items which contain ..., ... or ... should only be consumed in small amounts.

3 A nutrition hotline

23 Three people call the NHS Nutrition Hotline for advice about food. Listen and match the items below to the telephone calls.

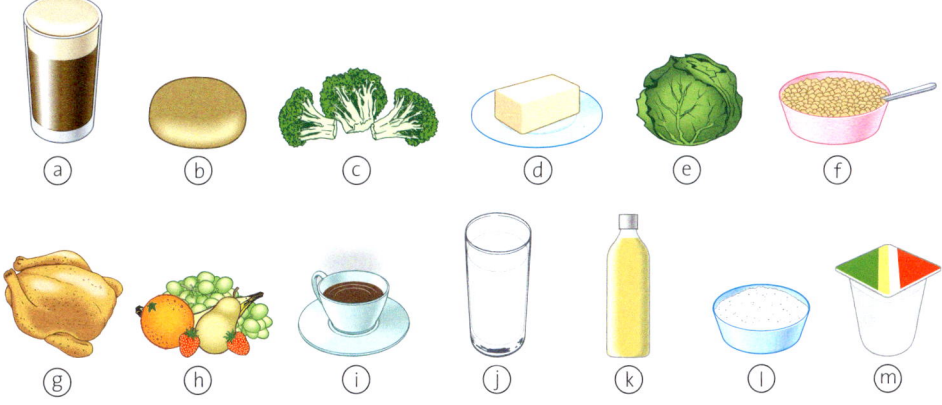

23 Now listen to the three calls again and say whether the following statements are true or false. Correct the false statements.

1 High-fibre foods are some of the healthiest during pregnancy.
2 Vitamin D can be more harmful than vitamin A.
3 Coconut oil is healthier than olive oil.
4 Rapeseed oil and canola oil are the same.
5 Sweet teas are worse for your teeth than unsweetened teas.
6 Teas sweetened with sugar are some of the most popular baby products.

4 Working with words

Match the words with the definitions.

1 diet
2 cholesterol
3 fibre
4 to recommend
5 foetus
6 to increase
7 harmful
8 to limit
9 cereals

a) to keep below a certain amount
b) to tell someone that something is good
c) breakfast food made from grains
d) to make something higher
e) part of food that passes through the body
f) what you eat
h) a young human or animal before birth
i) bad for you
g) a harmful substance in blood

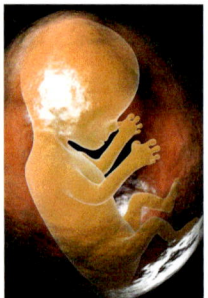

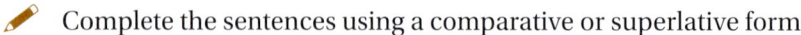

> **GRAMMAR CHECK** Comparatives and superlatives (Steigerung der Adjektive)
>
> 1 Some fruit teas are **sweeter** **than** the unsweetened teas.
> 2 Animal fat is **more harmful** **than** vegetable oil.
> 3 They are one of **the most popular** baby products.
> 4 Unsweetened teas are **better** for babies **than** sweet teas.
>
> - Die meisten einsilbigen Adjektive und alle zweisilbigen Adjektive mit den Endungen *-y*, *-er* und *-ow* werden mit *-(e)r, -(e)st* gesteigert (1).
> - Die meisten zweisilbigen und alle mehrsilbigen Adjektive werden mit *more/most, less/ least* gesteigert (2, 3).
> - Ausnahmen sind *good – better – best; bad – worse – worst* und *little – less – least* (4).

5 Practice

Complete the sentences using a comparative or superlative form.

1 Skimmed milk is ... (healthy) than full fat milk.
2 Saturated fats are the ... (dangerous) type of fats.
3 People with heart disease often have ... (high) cholesterol levels than normal.
4 Vitamin C and D are ... (good) for you than vitamin B.
5 Some fruit teas have ... (little) sugar in them than other sweetened teas.
6 Heart disease is one of the ... (big) killers in Europe.
7 Eating the right food is ... (important) than how much you eat.
8 Baby food in a jar is ... (quick) to prepare than fresh food.
9 A diet rich in folic acid is ... (good) for pregnant women.
10 Saturated fats are ... (harmful) than vegetable oils.
11 Bread and cereals are ... (high) in fibre than fruit.
12 Smoking is one of the ... (bad) things for a pregnant woman.
13 Is honey more or ... (harmful) for babies than sugar?
14 Acme medical insurance offers you the ... (good) treatment for the ... (little) cost.
15 Mr Castle's condition hasn't improved and is now ... (bad) than before.

6 A wordfield: Illness

Produce a list of all the words in the text that have something to do with illness.

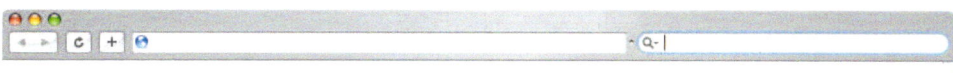

The truth about diabetes

With so much information about diabetes out there, be sure you're getting the correct facts. Here are some answers to some commonly asked questions.

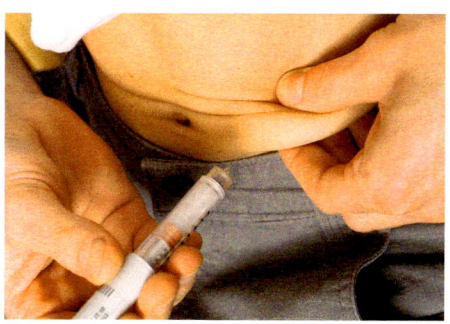

1 ...

Although we don't know why some people get diabetes, we know it is not contagious – it can't be caught like a cold or the flu.

2 ...

Diabetes is caused by a combination of genetic and environmental factors. However, a diet high in fat and sugar can cause you to become overweight. Being overweight increases your risk of developing Type 2 diabetes.

3 ...

There is no such thing as a mild form of diabetes. All diabetes is equally serious, and if not properly controlled can lead to serious health problems.

4 ...

If you have good control of your diabetes, research shows that people with diabetes are no less safe on the roads than anyone else. However, in the UK, people who treat their diabetes with insulin injections are not allowed to drive buses or coaches.

5 ...

Ask Steve Redgrave, the five-times Olympic gold medal-winning rower; or many of the other people with diabetes who take part in the London Marathon every year. People with diabetes should do exercise as part of a healthy lifestyle.

6 ...

You are not more likely to get a cold or another illness if you have diabetes. But people with diabetes are advised to get flu jabs. This is because any infection changes their blood glucose control, putting them at risk of high blood glucose levels.

7 ...

Sweets and other sugary foods are no more dangerous to people with diabetes than they are to the rest of us, if they're part of a healthy diet. Remember that confectionery foods are higher in fat and calories, too so for this reason you shouldn't eat too many, especially if you are trying to lose weight.

Diabetes

There are 2.5 million people in the UK with diabetes and more than half a million people who have the condition but don't know it.

7 Talking about diabetes

Match these questions with the paragraphs (1–7) in exercise 6.

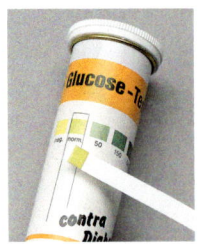

A Is it safe to drive if you have diabetes?
B Is it true people with diabetes shouldn't eat chocolate?
C Can eating too much sugar cause diabetes?
D Do people with diabetes get more colds and other illnesses?
E Is Type 2 the milder form of diabetes?
F Can I catch diabetes from someone else?
G Can I still play sport if I have diabetes?

8 Odd-one-out

Which word doesn't fit?

1 a) lead to   b) catch   c) cause
2 a) cold   b) diabetes   c) flu
3 a) environmental b) controlled   c) safe
4 a) diet   b) sport   c) exercise
5 a) genetic   b) contagious   c) infection
6 a) risk   b) danger   c) healthy
7 a) sugar   b) fibre   c) glucose
8 a) lifestyle   b) jabs   c) injections

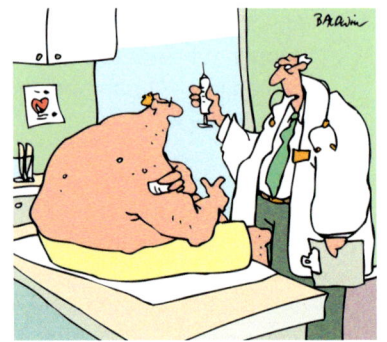

"It wasn't really Insulin. You don't have diabetes yet. It was just a warning shot."

9 Working with words

Complete the sentences with words from exercise 8.

1 A ... high in fat and sugar can make you overweight.
2 A good diet and exercise are part of a healthy ... .
3 Diabetes is not ... - you can't get it from other people like a cold.
4 If someone with diabetes gets the flu, it can cause high blood ... levels.
5 All forms of diabetes can ... serious health problems if not controlled.
6 People can be very active and still play ... if they have diabetes.
7 Catching ... can cause problems with blood glucose control.
8 For some people, their diabetes must be ... by insulin injections.

10 Controlling diabetes

Magda Jakimowicz is a patient with Type 2 diabetes. Listen to a medical assistant give her advice. Make notes in your exercise book about what the patient has to do.

What words are missing from Magda's treatment?

Magda must take ...[1] and change her ...[2]. She must keep to a healthy ...[3] and lose ...[4]. She must also monitor her blood ...[5] levels.

TV chef fights for healthier school dinners

New guidelines on school meals mark the latest victory for TV chef Jamie Oliver in his fight to introduce healthier eating habits into schools in England. Oliver started his *Feed Me Better* campaign because of the junk food being served in many English schools. His hit television programme *Jamie's School Dinners* saw him asking children to eat salads and fruit rather than chips and burgers. Schools also looked at banning crisps, confectionery and snacks as well as sugary and carbonated drinks from schools.

The television show, which had millions of viewers, reported that the average school dinner cost just 45p to make and led to the government giving an extra €300m to improve school dinners in England.

But despite the popularity of the award-winning TV show and the introduction of healthy school dinner guidelines, Oliver's fight is far from over. A recent report shows a 17% drop in the number of children eating school dinners since the healthy guidelines were introduced. Mr Curran, a director of care services, warns of a growing black market for non-nutritional foods and problems with burger vans outside school gates. 'I've seen chips being passed through school gates.' he added. 'Everyone wants to see healthy food in our schools, but if we're not careful it could destroy the service.'

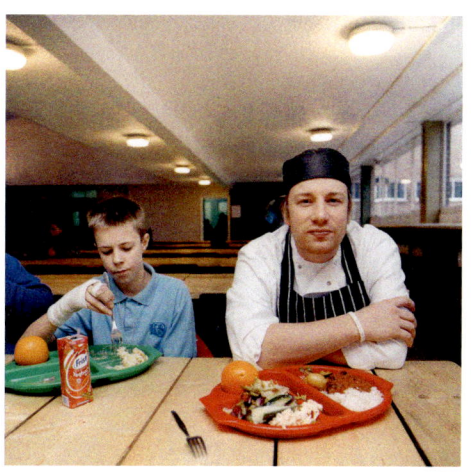

1 A discussion of pros and cons

Work with a partner. Student A reads the article again and makes notes on the positive effects of Jamie Oliver's campaign. Student B makes notes on the negative effects of the campaign.

Then discuss whether the campaign has been a success or not.

2 Working with words

Match the words and phrases (1–7) with the definitions (a–g).

1	guidelines	a)	say something must not be done
2	victory	b)	a drink with small bubbles
3	junk food	c)	instructions about the best way to do something
4	ban	d)	when something happens even when you try to stop it
5	carbonated	e)	success when you win something
6	despite	f)	damage something so badly it can't be used
7	destroy	g)	non-nutritional food full of fats and sugars

8 Dealing with illness

1 Seeing the doctor

T 25 Julia Michaels is an American woman working in Freiburg. She goes to see Dr Müller. Listen and write down Julia's symptoms. Then listen again and say which phrases (a–h) Dr Müller uses to reassure Julia.

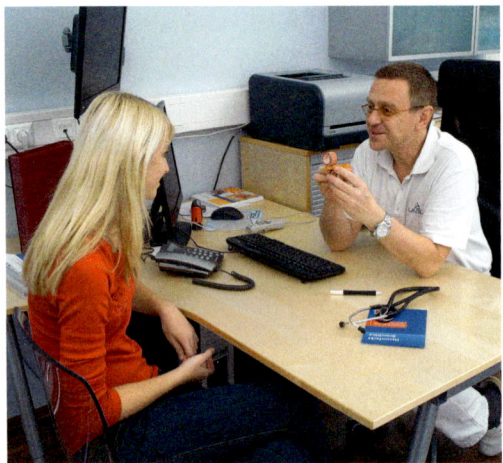

a) You shouldn't assume the worst, you know.
b) I'm sure there's nothing to worry about.
c) Sensations like that can be perfectly normal.
d) Don't worry about sensations like that.
e) But don't get all worried about …
f) I don't think you need to worry about …
g) Blood tests are normal.
h) Blood tests are very routine.

2 Practice

Match the words and phrases with a similar meaning.

1	strange	a)	weak
2	pins and needles	b)	weird
3	no energy	c)	dizzy
4	normal	d)	difficulties
5	problems	e)	depressed
6	lack of balance	f)	tingling feeling
7	really down	g)	routine

> **LANGUAGE** Reassuring patients
>
> I'm a bit worried about …
> There's nothing to worry about.
> Don't worry, it's just a …
> It's just a …, it won't hurt.
> It's a very routine operation/test.
> It's perfectly normal.

> **GRAMMAR CHECK** The going to future
>
> 1 I'm just **going to ask** you some questions.
> 2 **Are** you **going to use** a needle?
> 3 Don't worry, this **isn't going to hurt**.
>
> Die Struktur *am/is/are going to* + Grundform des Verbs wird verwendet, um über Absichten zu sprechen (1, 2), oder wenn die Gewissheit (oder ein Anzeichen dafür) besteht, dass etwas geschehen wird (3).

3 Practice

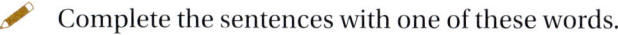 Complete the sentences with the 'going to' form of the verbs in brackets.

1 She ... (take) a blood sample.
2 It ...(not/be) very warm today.
3 ... you ...(give) me some medicine?
4 We ...(be) late if you don't hurry up.
5 I ...(study) hard for my English test.
6 You can already see he ...(be) a difficult patient.
7 It's very busy today. They ...(not/fit) everyone in before lunch.
8 ... she ...(see) the doctor?
9 I ...(refer) you to a neurologist.
10 ... my symptoms ...(get) worse?

4 Practice

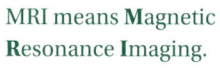 Complete the sentences with one of these words.

ankle | appendix | back | buttocks | chest | chin | elbow | hip | jaw | kidneys |
knee | liver | lungs | neck | shoulder | stomach | thigh | throat

1 He's going to have his ... examined as he's often short of breath.
2 A lot of office workers are going to have lower ... problems because of the way they sit.
3 I can't speak very well because I have a very sore ....
4 She's going to have an operation to take a stone out of her ....
5 I had a really bad pain in my side one day and had to go to hospital. They took my ... out the same day.
6 'Tennis ...' is a joint problem that affects more than just tennis players.
7 I'm going to have an operation on my ... because I can't bend my leg any more.
8 'Whiplash' is a ... condition often caused by car crashes.

5 An MRI scanner

What do you know about MRI scanners?
What can you find out on the Internet?

MRI means **M**agnetic **R**esonance **I**maging.

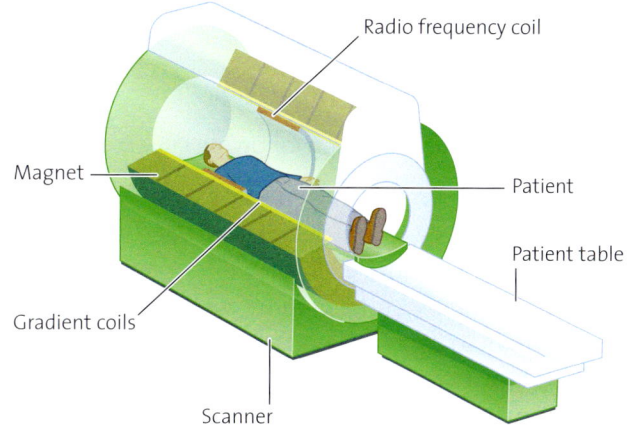

Radio frequency coil

Magnet

Patient

Patient table

Gradient coils

Scanner

6 An MRI scan

T 26 Julia Michaels goes for an MRI scan. Heike Völler is the technician preparing her for the scan. Listen, make notes and then explain what the procedure is.

Heike   Hello Ms Michaels. My name's Heike and I'm going to look after you today.

Julia   Hi. Nice to meet you.

Heike   Is this the first time you've had a scan?

Julia   Yes, it is. And I'm a little nervous.

Heike   No need to worry. The scanner is like a big camera and we're going to take some pictures of you. It's all very safe. Now, have you filled in the questionnaire?

Julia   Err, yes. Here it is.

Heike   Great. Thanks. OK, so this all looks good. So you have nothing metal in you at all? That's good! Now, I'm going to have to ask you to undress and put this gown on. And you need to take off everything that is metal, like your watch or any jewellery. And could you please take off your bra as it has metal clasps – we can't put anything metal in the scanner, you see.

Julia   Oh, OK.

Heike   That's great. Here let me help you with the gown. OK, now could you please lie back on the table? In a minute I'm going to move the table into the scanner and we can start scanning. The scanner can be a bit noisy, so put these earplugs in. That's it. And can I just put your head in between these pads here? That's perfect. And it can be a bit cold, so I'm just going to put a blanket over you. OK? Great. Now when the machine starts, it will make a loud banging noise for a minute or so and then go quiet for a few seconds, and then start again. The whole thing should last about 45 minutes. Are you comfortable?

Julia   Yes, thanks.

Heike   Good. Now I'm going to leave the room but don't worry, I'm going to keep talking to you and telling you what's happening. Right, let's get started!

Listen again and write down the reassuring language Heike uses in your exercise book.

7 Multiple Sclerosis facts

Work with a partner. Are the following statements about Multiple Sclerosis (MS) true or false?

1   No-one knows exactly what causes MS.
2   Old people are more likely to suffer from MS.
3   Multiple Sclerosis attacks more men than women.
4   Treatment to cure MS is very expensive.
5   Scientists are testing a new drug that can cure MS.

Now read the text on the opposite page quickly to check your answers.

New hope for Multiple Sclerosis sufferers

Doctors are not sure what causes it and there is no known cure. But for thousands of people whose lives are changed by MS, there is perhaps at last, hope for the future.

Multiple Sclerosis (MS) is a condition in which the immune system attacks the central nervous system and affects the transfer of messages to the rest of the body. The disease usually occurs in young adults and is more common in women. There is currently no cure, and treatment focuses on easing symptoms.

However, there is now hope on the horizon. Researchers at Bristol University say that their work will possibly – in the next ten years – lead to the development of new drugs that will be able to treat the disease.

The team found that mice with high levels of galanin, a protein in brain nerve cells, were not attacked by multiple sclerosis. Scientists already know that galanin helps protect the nervous system. When a nerve is injured, levels of galanin increase dramatically as the body limits cell death. Researchers have now proved that mice that are given high levels of galanin won't develop MS.

David Wynick, Professor at Bristol University said: 'We gave the mice MS and the results show that high levels of galanin in the mice protect them completely from MS – the disease won't attack them at all. In contrast, mice that had no galanin had much more severe cases of MS.'

The team now hopes it will produce a drug with the effects of galanin, which can be used to slow the progress of multiple sclerosis. It will take many years, but there is hope on the horizon.

Main symptoms of
Multiple sclerosis

Central:
• fatigue
• cognitive impairment
• depression
• unstable mood

Visual:
• nystagmus
• optic neuritis
• diplopia

Throat:
• dysphagia

Speech:
• dysarthria

Musculoskeletal:
• weakness
• spasms
• ataxia

Sensation:
• pain
• hypoesthesias
• paraesthesias

Bowel:
• incontinence
• diarrhoea or constipation

Urinary:
• incontinence
• frequency or retention

FACT FILE Multiple Sclerosis

There are 400,000 MS sufferers in the USA.
There are 90,000 sufferers in the UK.
The highest risk ages are 20–40 years old.
Whites are twice as likely to get MS than other races.
Women are twice as likely to get MS as men.

Answer the following questions.

1 What is Multiple Sclerosis?
2 What does treatment try to do?
3 What is galanin and why is it important?
4 When will the new drugs be ready?

8 Multiple Sclerosis symptoms

Work with a partner. Read the article again and look at the information about the symptoms of MS. With your partner think how these symptoms change people's lives. Think about work, hobbies and home life.

> **GRAMMAR CHECK** The will-future
>
> 1 New drugs that **will be able to** treat the disease.
> 2 Their work **will** possibly **lead to** the development of new drugs.
> 3 Mice that are given high levels of galanin **won't develop** MS.
>
> - Mit *will* (+ Grundform) werden Vorhersagen und Annahmen über die Zukunft ausge-drückt, auf die wir keinen Einfluss haben (1).
> - Das *will*-Futur wird oft im Zusammenhang mit Signalwörtern wie *think, maybe, possibly* oder *probably* benutzt (2).
> - Im gesprochenen English wird *will* meist abgekürzt. Beachte: *will not = won't* (3).

9 Practice

Complete the following sentences with the correct form of will.

1 Scientists ... (continue) to look for a cure for MS.
2 A cure ... (not/be) ready for many years yet.
3 When ... the new drugs ...(be) ready?
4 The drugs ... (help) slow down the progress of the disease.
5 An MS sufferer ... (need) to have regular appointments.
6 The disease ... (not/always/get) worse quickly.
7 What kind of tests ... I ...(have to) have?
8 When ... I ... (get) the results of the test?
9 The anaesthetic ... (take) a minute or two to work.
10 We ... (not/get) the results back until Thursday.

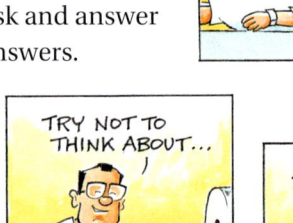

WHATEVER YOU DO...

10 Practice

Work with a partner. Take it in turns to ask and answer these questions. Give reasons for your answers.

1 Do you think there will be a cure for MS?
2 Do you think doctors will find out what causes MS?
3 Do you think we will find new diseases in the future?
4 Do you think one day doctors will be able to cure every disease?

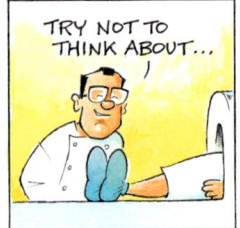

TRY NOT TO THINK ABOUT...

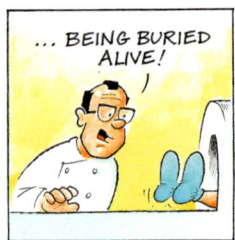

... BEING BURIED ALIVE!

11 Practice

Work with a partner. Look at the pictures below and say what you think is going to happen. Does your partner agree? Use these words.

blood sample | stethoscope | bank card | thermometer | examination | MRI scan

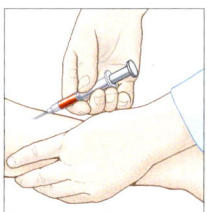 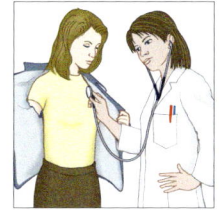

I think he/she is going to …

I don't agree.
It looks like …

Yes, I think so, too.

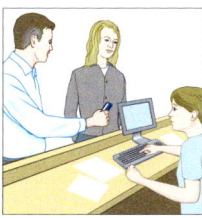 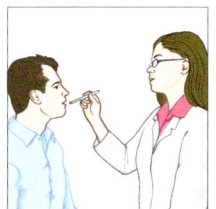 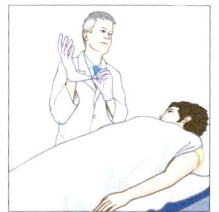 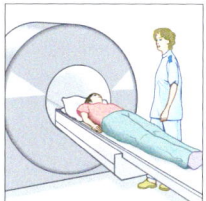

GRAMMAR CHECK Will-future or going to-future?

1 Doctor: **I'll have** your results next week. *(Annahme)*
2 Patient: **I'm going to ask** the doctor to change my medication. *(Absicht)*
3 Nurse: The doctor **will/is going to give** you the results next week.
4 Friend: **Are** you **going to/Will** you **ask** the doctor to change your medication?

Je nach Sprechabsicht wählt ein Sprecher eine der beiden Zukunftsformen (1, 2). Aber sind die Sprechabsichten unbekannt oder nicht erkennbar, sind beide Formen austauschbar (3, 4).

12 How MS progresses

Listen to a neurologist talk about the different forms of MS. Complete the text on the following page with the correct subtypes in the box below.

Primary-progressive MS
Secondary-progressive MS
Relapsing-remitting MS
Progressive-relapsing MS

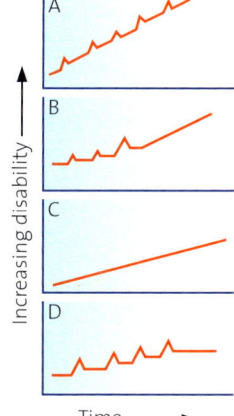

A Progressive-relapsing multiple sclerosis: steady decline since onset with superimposed attacks

B Secondary-progressive multiple sclerosis: initial relapsing-remitting multiple sclerosis that suddenly begins to have decline without periods of remission

C Primary-progressive multiple sclerosis: steady increase in disability without attacks

D Relapsing-remitting multiple sclerosis: unpredictable attacks which may or may not leave permanent deficits followed by periods of remission

Increasing disability →

Time →

The course of MS is difficult to predict. The disease can be dormant or progress steadily. Doctors use information about a patient's symptoms in the past to predict the future course of the disease. Today there are four recognized subtypes of MS.

1 ... This describes the early course of the disease for nearly 90% of sufferers. There are sudden attacks (relapses) followed by months or even years with no sign of the disease (remission).

2 ... About 80% of sufferers with relapsing-remitting MS then begin to have more frequent attacks without periods of remission in between. The patient declines steadily and new symptoms appear. This is the most common form of MS.

3 ... This describes about 10% of patients who never have periods of remission after the first signs of MS appear. Symptoms increase and the decline is steady. This subtype normally affects people who are older when the disease strikes.

4 ... This is the least common subtype and describes patients who show a steady decline but also suffer severe attacks at regular intervals.

13 Types of MS

Work with a partner. A South African woman comes to your hospital for an MRI scan. Act a dialogue between the technician and the patient.

Technician	Patient
Greet and reassure patient.	
	Greet technician.
Ask if patient has completed questionnaire.	
	Hand over completed questionnaire.
Ask patient to undress and explain why it is necessary.	
	Ask technician to explain what is going to happen.
Reassure patient and explain what the procedure is.	
	Ask questions about anything you don't understand.
Answer questions and reassure the patient.	

Extra material

1 The human side

Read the case study from an MS website. Then make notes in your exercise book under the following headings.

Type of MS	How diagnosed	Current treatment

My Life with MS by Steven May

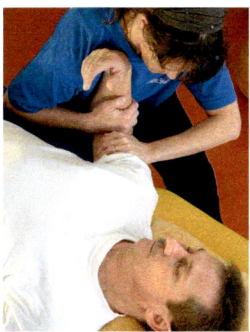

I was diagnosed with relapsing remitting multiple sclerosis in March 2004 at the age of 25. Before then I was a fit man with a successful career and a very active long-distance runner.

My story really begins one morning, when I woke up with a numb right thigh. I carried on as normal but after a week of no feeling in my right leg I went to see my GP. He quickly sent me to see a specialist and I underwent lots of tests including an MRI scan and a lumbar puncture. The numbness continued to get worse and moved into other parts of my body.

The following week I returned to see my neurologist and was diagnosed with MS, which I knew nothing about at the time. I quickly researched my condition, began lots of physiotherapy and started to fight back.

My condition changed a lot during the first couple of years and I experienced new and varied medication during that time. As well as still doing lots of physiotherapy every day, I have to take a cocktail of tablets. Life with MS is varied. I have constant problems that are always there but new issues appear all the time. I get on and deal with each new problem as it arises. I get on with my life with a positive outlook and look for the best, not the worst life has to throw at me.

As the years have gone by, my MS has altered the way I live my life, but has also opened doors and allowed me to experience new things and meet people I would not have met in my old life. Although I have left my old job, I am too young to retire and I am studying for a new career. I am the secretary for the local MS Society and I'm working for the MS support centre. I have three children to keep me active and a supportive partner who I could not be without. I have MS, but it does not have me.

2 Looking deeper

What do you think the author means by the following statements?

1 'I started to fight back' (paragraph 3)
2 'I get on and deal with each new problem' (paragraph 4)
3 'MS has opened doors' (paragraph 5)
4 'I have MS but it doesn't have me.' (final line)

1 Eating disorders

Work with a partner. Read the e-mail to a magazine advice column and choose the correct answer for each question. Do you and your partner agree?

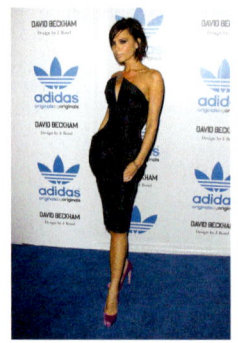

Dear Carrie
My friend seems to be getting thinner and thinner, but she eats a lot. I don't know what's wrong with her. But she never wants to talk about it. What can I do? How can I help her? I'm very worried about her.   *Petra K.*

1   How do eating disorders start?
   a) It's genetic. You get it from your parents.
   b) They are caused by mental illness.
   c) Because of all the women's magazines.

2   What other symptoms might Petra's friend show?
   a) Depression, no energy, anxiety about everything
   b) Obsession with food, her looks and her weight
   c) Bad stomach pains and regular sickness

3   Carrie should advise Petra to tell her friend to …
   a) stop being stupid and eat something.
   b) think about her parents and family.
   c) talk to someone she trusts and see a doctor.

FACT FILE Eating disorders

- Obesity kills 35,000 people a year in the UK. You are obese if you have a **B**ody **M**ass **I**ndex (weight in kilograms divided by the square of your height in metres) of 30 or more.
- About 165,000 people in the UK suffer from eating disorders. 1 in 10 are men. Eating disorders kill around 19,000 people a year in the UK.

2 Symptoms of eating disorders

T 28   Listen to this radio interview with a health expert. Match the symptoms to the disorders.

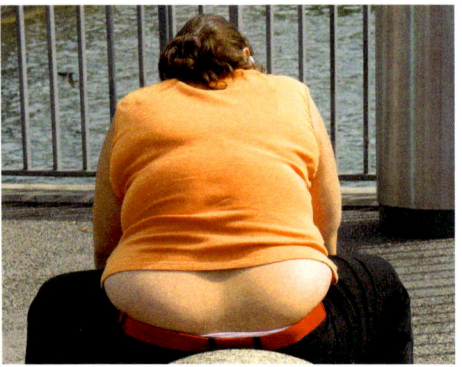

Eating disorders: 1. anorexia nervosa | 2. bulimia | 3. overeating

Symptoms: a) depression | b) fast or irregular heart rate | c) dental problems | d) low blood pressure | e) poor circulation | f) purging/controlled vomiting | g) frequent headaches | h) bingeing | i) hair growth on face | j) no energy or enthusiasm | k) feeling cold | l) high blood pressure

3 Dealing with eating disorders

 Read the text below and match the headings (a–e) to the paragraphs 1–5.

a) Provide a healthy family environment | b) Be sensitive to their emotions | c) Ask for professional help | d) Encourage their creative abilities | e) Don't ignore the signs

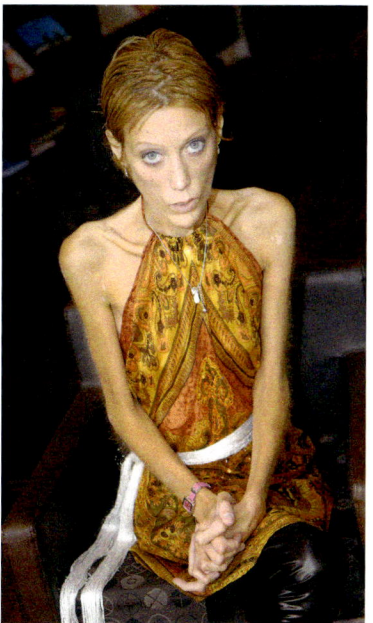

Teenage Eating Disorders – What can the family do?

Statistics show that about 10% of the U.S. population suffers from some form of eating disorder. Almost 95% of sufferers are women, most of them aged between 10 and 20. For families who have teenagers suffering from these disorders, here are the steps that can be taken to address the problem before it gets worse.

1 ...

Treatment clinics for people suffering from eating problems can be found everywhere. These facilities generally offer psychological counselling, nutritional therapy and medical attention.

2 ...

If you think that your adolescent child is just picky with his or her food, you might miss the chance to treat the disorder when it starts, which is always the best time to deal with the problem. Look for symptoms, like being too worried about body weight, obsession with counting calories and weighing food, uncontrolled eating or dieting, vomiting or purging and extreme mood swings.

3 ...

Eating disorders can start because of a traumatic experience. Experts say that some people who suffer from one of these disorders have been abused as a child. Teenage girls and boys who have experienced failure and humiliation also sometimes turn to overeating or not eating at all as a way of dealing with their emotions.

4 ...

Don't try to avoid family problems. If there are big changes within the family that can hurt your teenager, talk about it in the open and try to get them to talk about their feelings and say what they think about the situation. However, don't be too pushy as this is something that teenagers really don't like.

5 ...

Letting teenagers do activities that they like and they are good at can give them a good emotional and psychological foundation. Encourage them to express their thoughts and ideas and do their hobbies, but don't make them live up to your personal expectations of them. Teenage eating disorders are not just physical health problems, they are primarily psychological and should be addressed by giving young people all the love and support that they need.

4 Odd-one-out

Which word doesn't fit?

	a)		b)		c)
1	address		deal with		offer
2	population		adolescent		teenager
3	abused		overweight		misused
4	failure		treatment centres		clinics
5	counselling		support		statistics
6	express		expectation		talk
7	depressed		pushy		mood swings
8	symptoms		obsession		uncontrolled

5 Working with words

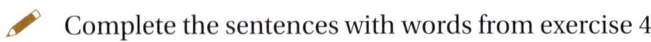

Complete the sentences with words from exercise 4.

1 A professional counselor should ... problems to do with eating disorders.
2 The majority of cases are ... girls aged between 10-20 years old.
3 Some experts think eating disorders start when children are ... .
4 There are many ... where people with eating disorders can get help.
5 Many disorders are emotional and can be treated by psychological ... .
6 People with eating problems often feel unable to ... their thoughts and feelings.
7 Teenagers don't like it when parents are ... and make them do things.
8 An early sign is an unhealthy ... with looks and weight.

6 A growing weight problem

T 29 Listen to an expert from the US National Obesity Forum explain why so many young people are overweight.

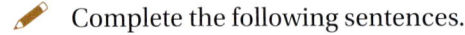

Complete the following sentences.

1 Kids in the USA are becoming ... .
2 People are obese when their ... is 30 or more.
3 Kids today do far less physical ... .
4 They also eat less ... food.
5 Kids copy each other's eating ... .
6 Obesity inreases the risk of type 2 ... .
7 More than ... Americans have diabetes.

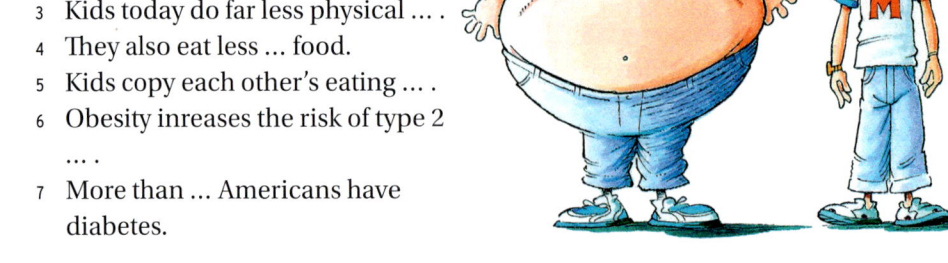

T 29 Listen again and say what the following numbers refer to.

a) 10–17   b) 49   c) 30   d) 18–25   e) 37%   f) 150bn

7 Psychological problems

 Why shouldn't you say any of the things below to someone with an eating disorder? Read the article below and match 1-7 to the psychological problems (a–d).

1. Why are you doing this to me? | 2. Are you sick? | 3. I don't understand how you can eat so much. | 4. You look like you've got AIDS. | 5. If you love your family, eat something. | 6. You'll make yourself sick if you don't eat. | 7. That's why you haven't got many friends.

Eating disorders and the mind

People who suffer from eating disorders DO NOT need to look underweight or act differently. Many men and women have normal body weight but can still suffer badly from any of these psychological problems.

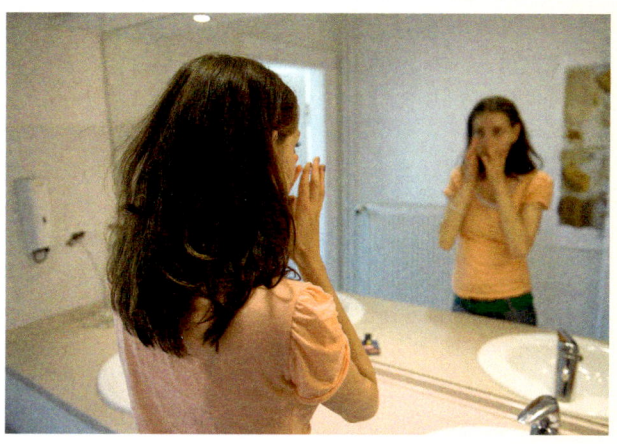

a) Negative self-image

This includes feelings such as 'I never do anything right' or 'people will like me more if I lose weight.' Anorexics and bulimics often want everything to be perfect and they starve themselves or binge if they don't do things well. Overeaters are often called 'fat' or 'lazy', which makes them feel very lonely.

b) Guilt

People with eating disorders often worry about all of the problems they give their friends and family. They feel bad about not being a 'strong and normal person' and find it hard to meet the expectations of parents and friends.

c) Power

Anorexics and bulimics often experience highs after a binge. They think they are still in control of the problem if they can carefully plan their binges and purges. This feeling of control is all they have and they fight people who try to take it away from them.

d) Depression

This includes low motivation, feelings of hopelessness, worrying about everything and feeling completely alone. In some cases depression can even lead to people with eating disorders taking their own lives.

8 Working with words

 Choose the correct word to complete the sentences.

1. Anorexics don't always look badly underweight/overweight.
2. Many eating disorders are caused by psychological/mind problems.
3. Anorexics can binge/starve themselves if things don't go well.
4. Overweight people are often called lonely/lazy.
5. Bulimics can experience highs/purges like a drug user.
6. They often feel guilty/alone about the problems they cause.

GRAMMAR CHECK If-Clauses type 1 (If-Sätze)

1. People **will like** me more if I **lose** weight.
2. Sufferers **can die** if they **don't respond** to treatment.
3. They **are** still in control if they **can** carefully **plan** their binges.
4. If you **love** your family, **eat** something.

- *If-clauses* vom Typ 1: *If*-Satz mit *simple present* – Hauptsatz mit *will* + Verb. (1)
- Im Hauptsatz können anstelle von *will* andere Modalverben wie *can* (2), eine Gegenwartsform von *be* (3) und Verben in der Befehlsform (4) stehen.

---

9 Practice

Complete the following sentences with the correct form of the verbs.

1. If you ... (be) worried about someone's eating, ... (speak) to a doctor.
2. Sometimes anorexics ... (starve) themselves if things ... (not/go) well.
3. Children ... (be) more likely to be obese if they ... (have) overweight friends.
4. Teenagers ... (not/like) it if parents ... (be) too pushy.
5. If you ... (not/notice) the symptoms early, the problem ... (get) worse.
6. If there ... (be) changes in the family, ... (talk) about them with your child.
7. Teenagers ... (feel) guilty if they ... (think) they're causing problems.
8. You ... (be) clinically obese if your BMI ... (be) higher than 30.
9. You ... (see) a doctor if you ... (think) you have problems with food.

10 Internet research

Find the information you need to match the foods (1–10) with the number of calories per 100 grams (a–j).

1. butter | 2. fried egg | 3. boiled egg | 4. whole milk | 5. skimmed milk | 6. bacon | 7. grilled beef steak | 8. apricot | 9. date | 10. brazil nut

a) 28 | b) 35 | c) 66 | d) 160 | e) 239 | f) 248 | g) 300 | h) 600 | i) 644 | j) 770

11 Failure to thrive

Katja is a medical assistant at a small practice. A foreign woman walks in with a small child. Complete the dialogue with the sentences below.

a) Don't worry, I'm sure the doctor will be able to help you. | **b)** What's the problem? |
c) I can understand why you're so worried. | **d)** I'm sorry to hear that. | **e)** Do you have an appointment? | **f)** I see what you mean.

Patient Good morning. Do you speak English?

Katja Yes, I do. Can I help you?

Patient Yes, I need to see a doctor about my child.

Katja ...¹

Patient No, not here. I have an appointment with a specialist in three weeks, but I need to see a doctor now.

Katja ...²

Patient My son isn't eating enough and he's losing weight.

Katja ...³

Patient I don't know what to do and I'm really worried.

Katja Hmm. ...⁴ I'll make an emergency appointment for you.
...⁵ Do you mind waiting an hour or so?

Patient Oh, I hope it won't take too long. My son looks so underweight.

Katja ...⁶ But he looks alert and healthy, so I'm sure he'll be OK.

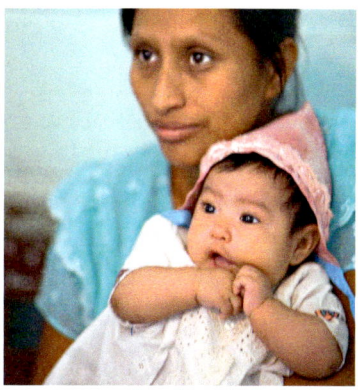

12 Showing sympathy

Work with a partner to make a dialogue.

Medical assistant	Patient
Greet new person and ask if you can help.	Ask if assistant can speak English.
Say you can and ask if he/she has an appointment.	Say no and ask if you can see the doctor.
Ask what the problem is.	Say what is wrong with you and why you need to see the doctor now.
Show sympathy and offer an emergency appointment.	Thank the assistant and say you can wait.

1 Super slim me

After the introduction, the following paragraphs in the article are mixed up. Read each one carefully and then put them in the correct order.

Super slim me

Despite young women starving themselves to death, the catwalks at London Fashion Week are still full of size zero models. TV presenter Dawn Porter finds out what life on a 'zero diet' is really like.

a) …

'But then a terrible thing started to happen. As the weight fell off me, I really liked how I looked. For the first time, my tummy was flat. Even though I was always hungry, I was excited to see how much more I could lose. I cut back to 400 calories a day – even going as low as 250 calories on some days. Suddenly I understood the madness of pro-anorexia websites and the results of starvation.'

b) …

At the start of the challenge, Dawn weighed 63kg with a BMI of 22 – which was the perfect weight for her height. 'When I took on the challenge of a starvation diet, I thought that hunger would be my biggest problem. The hunger actually became a sick comfort to me as the hungrier I was, the more I felt I was doing the right thing. I was on 500 calories a day and obsessing about what I was eating. I soon started to feel tired all the time as I couldn't sleep at night because of the permanent hunger.'

c) …

Then my doctor advised me to stop. My mineral levels were dangerously low and I risked my periods stopping and my hair growing thin. I was suffering headaches and terrible constipation and my immune system was so weak I risked infection. My BMI was down to 18 and my dress size a UK 8, but my life was no better, or more successful than before. I'd never felt so unattractive and it was the worst time of my life.'

d) …

In August 2006, 22-year-old Uruguayan model Luisel Ramos died after starving herself. She had tried to live on nothing but cola and lettuce leaves for three months. At the time of her death she had a BMI of 14.5. The World Health Organization considers a BMI of below 16 to be starvation. Six months later, her sister Eliana Ramos, 18, was found dead in her bedroom. She, too, had worked as a model and died of malnutrition and anorexia.

e) …

But for all my joy of losing weight, by week seven the depression kicked in. I'd never suffered depression in my life, but suddenly I would cry for no reason. Even though I'd never looked so slim, I was more insecure about my body than ever before. I felt unattractive. I went out on a date, but it was a disaster because I talked about dieting and calories all night. Men didn't find me attractive and women were jealous of my thinness.

f) …

In order to find out exactly what young models such as the Ramos sisters must go through to become a size zero, TV presenter Dawn Porter went on a crash diet. For two months a film crew recorded her as she tried to go from a curvy UK size 12 to a super skinny size 4 (US size zero). 'My aim was to show what kind of a miserable life you have to lead, what food you must eat – or must not eat – and the exercise you must do if you want to be a size zero.'

2 Paragraph summaries

Match the summaries (1–6) to the paragraphs (a–f).

1 Dawn's normal body size
2 Why she had to stop the diet
3 Introduction to the problem
4 Why young women follow the zero diet
5 How the diet changed Dawn's life
6 Why Dawn accepted the challenge

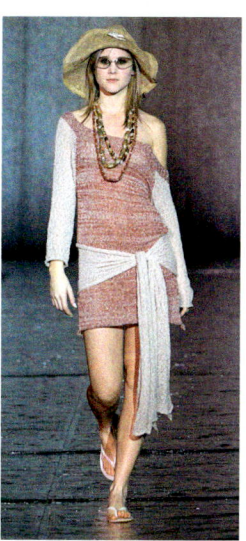

FACT FILE dreams and reality

- 6% of women are underweight, but 44% are overweight.
- Around 40% of models have an eating disorder.
- In 2006, Madrid Fashion Week banned size zero models.

3 Working with words

Choose the correct words from the box to complete each sentence.

anorexia | challenge | curvy | cut back | depressed | depression | disaster | hungry |
immune | insecure | jealous | kicked in | madness | malnutrition | obsessing | per-
manent | sick | skinny | starvation | tired | unattractive

1 When talking with friends, I was always ... about food.
2 When I reached size 8, friends started to say I looked ...
3 I couldn't sleep because of the ... hunger.
4 At less than 500 calories a day I was on a ... diet.
5 After a few weeks the depression ...
6 I obsessed about food and was ... about how I looked.
7 Many women are ... of other women who are slim.
8 Despite losing weight I felt ...
9 I thought the biggest ... would be the hunger.
10 I felt ... all the time because I couldn't sleep.
11 I understood how websites could be positive about ...
12 The World Health Organization says a BMI below 16 is ...

4 Mediation: Eating disorders

Your practice has a website and your boss has asked you to produce a webpage with the title 'What parents should know about eating disorders'. Look at all the information in the unit and produce an illustrated guideline. Give advice on how to spot eating disorders and how to deal with them. Can you provide links to some national and international organizations that help sufferers of eating disorders and offer advice and support to their families?

Applying for a job

1 The right person for the job

Work with a partner. Decide which characteristics are important for the three jobs below.

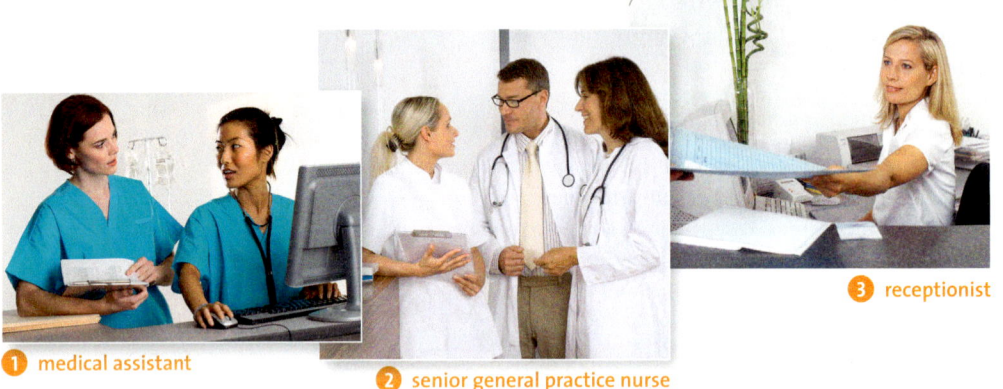

1 medical assistant

2 senior general practice nurse

3 receptionist

reliable | confident | friendly | strong | talkative | quiet | cheerful | able to keep calm | a good listener | well-organized | highly-qualified | responsible | accurate

I think a medical assistant/... should be ...

I agree. She/He should also be ...

A ... must always be ...

I don't think a senior general practice nurse needs to be ...

Perhaps, but he/she should be ...

2 What do you like or dislike about your job?

I like	working	overtime/weekends.
I enjoy	working with	alone.
I prefer	taking	stress.
...	dealing with	a friendly/unfriendly team.
	helping	samples of urine/blood.
I don't like/dislike	treating	(rude/unfriendly) patients.
I hate	using	our computer program.
I can't stand	giving	loud children.
...	...	...

I think ... is wonderful.

I think ... is terrible!

NVQs	(National Vocational Qualifications) These are vocational qualifications that can be assessed at level 2 or 3. They are gained at college, night school or by self-study while working. They can be taken at any age and are normally 9–18 months long courses.
RN	(Registered Nurse) A 3-year full-time course leading to a qualification approved by the Nursing and Midwifery Council (NMC).
FD	(Foundation Degree) A 2–3 year part-time, work-based learning programme at a university or college. The same as a university degree.
RCN	(Royal College of Nursing) The largest membership organization for nurses in the UK with over 395,000 members.
GPN	General Practice Nurse

3 Job advertisements

Make a table with five columns in an exercise book. The headings of the columns are: 1. Position, 2. Duties, 3. Qualifications, 4. Skills, 5. Other requirements. Now fill in the information from these job adverts from a British local newspaper.

1 Senior Receptionist

You will be responsible for organizing our reception team. This will include work routines and dealing with both patients and staff. Minimum 5 years' experience working on reception + qualifications required. You have good organizational skills, enjoy hard work and working with a strong team. Apply to Ms Emma Trow, Nuffield House Surgery, The Meadows, Harlow, CM8 4TP.

2 Grade E Experienced Staff Nurse

Registered nurse with a minimum of three years experience and assessment skills. Previous experience of disability assessment and experience of clinical decision-making. IT skills with experience of using a range of software (ECDL desirable). Highly developed written and verbal communication skills and evidence of ongoing professional development. Ability to work to targets and specified standards. Apply to Charles Davenport, Histon Medical Centre, Histon House, Harlow, CM15 7UU.

3 Care Assistant

Orchard House Retirement Village requires someone with good inter-personal skills to look after elderly people. Applicants must be smart, reliable and enthusiastic about caring for people. Experience required. Apply in writing to: Sarah Mason, Orchard House, High Wych Road, Sawbridgeworth, CM21 0GH

4 Hatfield Nursing Home

We are looking for a Home Care Assistant who is 17+ with some experience of care. Applicant will look after disabled people and do NVQ Level 2 training. Must have good people skills. Please apply in writing to: The Manager, Hatfield Nursing Home, Chaucer Way, Hatfield, A10 6LZ.

5 Receptionist *Termin verjeber*

Old Harlow Health Centre requires a receptionist for its small administration team. You will handle all inquiries, manage records and deal with patients in the waiting room. Applicants should have good communication skills, experience and good knowledge of reception software including 'Choose and book'. Apply in writing to Mrs Kathryn Lee, Old Harlow Health Centre, Terrace Gardens, Harlow, CM18 7TQ.

4 Looking for work

T 30 Listen to four young people describe themselves. Which of the jobs on the previous page do you think they should apply for?

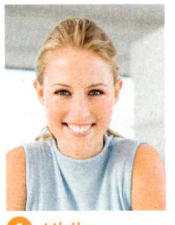

1 Ulrike

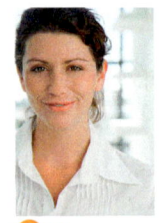

2 Sharon

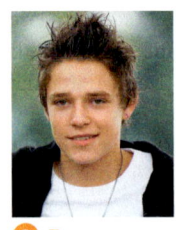

3 Tom

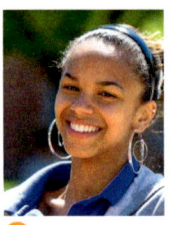

4 Kate

I think ... should apply for the job as a ... because ...

5 A letter of application

Complete Ulrike's letter of application with the phrases (a–h) below.

```
Dear Mrs Lee

...¹ the position of receptionist, which was advertised in the
Hertfordshire Evening News of 2 June.

...² a shop assistant in a large department store in Harlow. ...³
dealing with customers, offering product advice and achieving sales
targets.

As you can see from my enclosed CV, ...⁴ a doctor's assistant in
Germany before I married and moved to the UK with my British husband.
After six months I started work at John Lewis department store, where
I have worked since 2008. At John Lewis ...⁵ dealing with customers
in an English-speaking environment.

What interested me about your advertisement was the chance to work
in a small team, use some of the skills I learned during my three-year
training as a doctor's assistant and to learn new skills as part of
a career. I enjoy organizing information and I have excellent communi-
cation skills. ...⁶ computers.

...⁷ interview immediately. ...⁸ hearing from you soon.

Yours sincerely
Ulrike Morris

enc.
```

a I trained as	d I am currently working as	g I look forward to
b I am also good with	e I have gained experience in	h My duties include
c I would like to apply for	f I am available for	

6 Your Curriculum Vitae (CV)

Work with a partner. Make a list of all the things you should include in a good CV.

7 Writing a CV

Read the article from a U. S. website and match the headings with the paragraphs.

a) Education and professional qualifications

b) Summary

c) First impressions

d) Work experience

e) Length of CV

f) Personal details

g) Other experience

HOW TO WRITE THE KILLER CV

Your CV is a very important document; with it rest your hopes and dreams for the future – that next step up the career ladder, more money and new challenges. Your CV therefore has to represent the best you have to offer if you do not want to miss out on that perfect job you saw.

❶ ...

Your CV needs to attract the reader's attention in the first 20–30 seconds. An employer may have hundreds of CVs to look through. What an employer really wants to know is why they should invite you for an interview. If people cannot find what they want quickly, they will move on to someone else's CV. You should use appropriate headings and section breaks. Never send a hand-written CV or use a typewriter as you will look old fashioned and out of date.

❷ ...

It is usually best to try and keep your CV to two pages of A4. If you cannot keep your CV to this length, then you probably have not understood an employer's requirements. Employers do not want to know your whole life history – just enough to decide whether they should interview you or not.

❸ ...

Give your full name, address, home telephone number and mobile phone number. In the USA you don't need to include date of birth or marital status. You may want to include nationality if you are applying for jobs abroad.

❹ ...

List your education history, your professional qualifications, membership of professional associations and professional ID numbers. If you have recently completed a college or university degree or Diploma, etc, then you may want to list the courses you studied if the subject you studied was relevant to your target job.

❺ ...

Start with your most recent or last job and work backwards. Set out your main responsibilities, achievements, duties and skills that could be transferred to another employer. List your major achievements as an employer will only invite you for an interview if they can see a benefit in doing so.

❻ ...

List any computer skills you have and any foreign language skills which may be relevant for any jobs which you are applying for. Please list them and indicate whether your skills are spoken, written, business or technical.

❼ ...

List your major skills, strengths, personal qualities and achievements. Be specific, e.g. good team player, excellent written skills, versatile, able to motivate others, etc. Look at your staff appraisals or at your references.

What suggestions do you find surprising?

8 A Curriculum Vitae (CV)

🖉 Complete Ulrike's CV with the headings below.

Qualifications | Education | Address | Date of Birth | Work Experience |
Interests | Marital Status | Nationality | Additional Information

Name:	Ulrike Morris
❶ ...	8 Cedar Tree Lane, Torquay TQ1 4TR, Devon
Telephone	01279 8968702
E-mail	ulrikem2@hmail.com
❷ ...	5 August 1986
❸ ...	German
❹ ...	Married

❺ ...	2003–2005 Berufschule W4 (technical college) Hamburg, Germany 1997–2003 Erich Kästner Gesamtschule (comprehensive school) Hamburg
❻ ...	German equivalent of British GCSEs German qualification as doctor's assistant

❼ ... **2007–present   Shop assistant, John Lewis, Harlow**
Duties include dealing with customers, advising customers about products and helping the team achieve sales targets. I am also responsible for the presentation of the sales area and for managing stock levels.

2003–2006   Berufschule W4, Hamburg
Three-years' work experience as a doctor's assistant in a small private practice with sandwich release for study. I passed my exams in July 2006.

❽ ... I like listening to music and going out to the theatre and cinema. I also really enjoy travelling and seeing new places.

❾ ... I am a native German speaker and fluent in English. I also speak intermediate French and have excellent computer skills. I have a full European driving licence.

9 Content

Now read Ulrike's CV again and answer these questions.

1 Where is Ulrike working now?
2 When did she start working there?
3 What are her duties?
4 What exams did she take at school?

5 Where did she do her training?
6 What work experience does she have?
7 What skills does she have?
8 What are her interests and hobbies?

1 I **married** and moved to the UK.
2 I **passed** my exams in July 2004.
3 I **started** work at a department store, where I **have worked** since 2005.
4 Ulrike **has attached** her CV.

- Im *simple past* wird ein in der Vergangenheit vollständig abgeschlossener Vorgang geschildert (1, 2). Es wird häufig mit einer Zeitangabe der Vergangenheit (*yesterday, last week, ago, in 2002,* usw.) verwendet (2).
- Das *present perfect* wird verwendet, um auszudrücken, dass ein in der Vergangenheit begonnener Vorgang noch andauert (3), oder wenn etwas in der Vergangenheit geschehen ist, das noch Auswirkungen auf die Gegenwart hat (4).

10 Practice

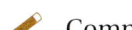

Complete the sentences about Ulrike with the simple past or present perfect.

1 Ulrike (leave) ... school in 2001.
   Ulrike **left** school in 2001.
2 After school she (train) ... as a doctor's assistant.
3 She (not/work) ... for very long in Germany.
4 She (go) ... to a comprehensive school in Hamburg.
5 She (pass) ... her driving test.
6 She (gain) ... a lot of experience in her present job.
7 She (come) ... to the UK in October 2005.
8 She (learn) ... how to speak English very well.

9 She (not/go) ... to school in England.
10 She (move) ... to the UK with her British husband.
11 She (apply) ... for a job in Harlow.
12 She (not/have) ... a reply from the practice yet.

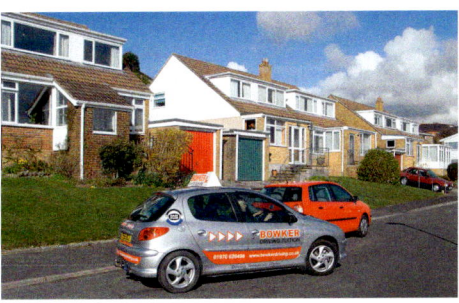

11 Writing your CV

Work with a partner. Look at the exercises on page 74 again. Then work together to write a CV for each of you.

Where do you work now?
How long have you been there?

When did you start working there?

I work for a small local practice called ... . How about you?

I started in ...

12 Preparing for an interview

T 31 Listen to a careers advisor's tips about how to prepare for a job interview.

Which of the following recommendations does the advisor give?

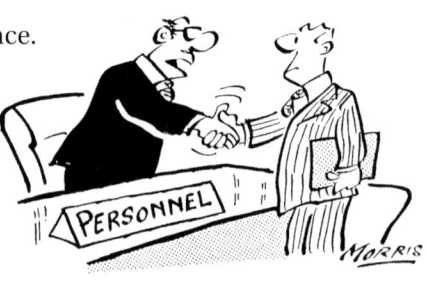

"I'll be in touch if we need somebody with integrity."

a) Start preparing for the interview well in advance.
b) Find out about the company on the internet.
c) Make friends with people who work for the company.
d) Always drive to the interview.
e) Change your CV to match the advertisement.
f) Practise the interview with a friend and record it.
g) Buy new clothes for the interview.
h) Look sexy – it might help you get the job.
i) Have a relaxing bath on the day of the interview.
j) Drink lots of coffee to stay awake.

13 Interview questions

Work with a partner. Make interview questions and answer them.

1	where / work / at the moment	I'm working at a practice in …
2	long / work / there	I've been with the practice for/since …
3	what / duties / include	I'm responsible for …
4	what / qualifications / have	I got my NVQ level 2/… in …
5	where / study	I went to … for three years then I …
6	what / hobbies and interests	I really like dancing/skydiving and …
7	what / enjoy / most / about /job	The thing I enjoy most about my job is …
8	what / strengths and weaknesses	I'm good at …, but I'm not so good at …
9	why / interested in / this job	What really interested me was the …
10	what / relevant skills / have	My English is very good and I can …
11	how / describe / yourself	I'm someone who can …

> **LANGUAGE** -er and -ee words
>
> employer – employee | interviewer – interviewee | trainer – trainee

14 Work with a partner

Work with a partner to prepare a job interview role-play.

- First choose one of the jobs from exercise 3 or find one on the Internet in English.
- Student A is the interviewer: Prepare some questions for the candidate.
- Student B is the interviewee: Use your CV from exercise 11.

1 Working in the UK

Ulrike got the job as a receptionist and is now working at a health centre in Harlow. She is talking to a friend about the problems of working in another country. List the things which are similar and the things which are different about training in the UK and in Germany.

How easy was it to get a job in the UK?

Very hard! I moved here with my British husband and then had to find a job. I sent my CV to everyone – pubs, retail – it took me six months of applying for jobs and having interviews before I got my first job at a department store. The worst thing was the interviews – I only had school English when I came to England, so the interviews were nerve-racking!

And how did you become a receptionist?

I saw the advertisement for a receptionist and applied. I had an interview with the owner and then I talked to the girls who work here and it just looked like a really nice place to work. And now I absolutely love it. But I want to get back into the clinical side of

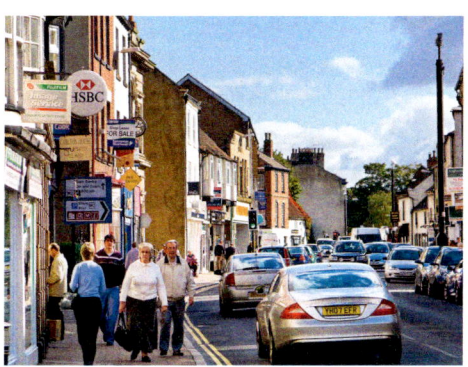

general practice so I'm doing some nursing training.

What is the training like in the UK?

It's great. I'm doing a two-year course and it's an NVQ Level 2 in general practice nursing. Because of my German qualifications I can do so many hours' clinical work but I still need to pass my British exams to be a qualified nurse and able to register with the Royal College of Nursing.

Is training in the UK very different from the training you did in Germany?

Yes and no. The clinical procedures are the same. But in Germany, as a trainee, I always felt I had no say in things and I had a senior nurse looking over my shoulder all the time. Here in the UK you get good pay and you get asked about changes to the practice and what you think about things.

And how do you like your job?

I absolutely love it! Every day is different and you never know what to expect.

And your future plans?

After I've qualified, I'd like to work full time on the clinical side and not reception. Then I'd like to do a degree I think.

2 About you

Write about the first week or so in your present job and about your plans for the future.

Transcripts

(N = narrator, M = man, W = woman)

Track 2: Unit 1, Ex. 1: At reception

Kerstin Guten Tag.

Gareth Ah, hello. Can you speak English?

Kerstin Yes, can I help you?

Gareth Yes. My name's Jones. Mr Gareth Jones. I've got an appointment.

Kerstin Mr Jones ... Ah, yes, the appointment was for ten thirty. But don't worry.

Gareth Oh, I am sorry. What time is it?

Kerstin It's twenty to eleven, but we aren't very busy today. We can fit you in.

Gareth Oh good. Thank you. Sorry.

Kerstin It's OK. Have you got your health insurance card with you?

Gareth Yes, I have. Here it is.

Kerstin And have you got ten euros for the surgery charge, please?

Gareth Yes, here you are.

Kerstin Thank you. And here's your receipt.

Gareth Thanks.

Kerstin: You're welcome. Please take a seat in the waiting room.

Gareth OK. Thank you.

Track 3: Unit 1, Ex. 3: What time is it?

N Phone call number 1.

W So, your appointment's on Wednesday at eleven thirty, Mrs Nicholl. That's half past eleven on the 25 June.

N Phone call number 2.

W That's right, Mrs Hanson, your appointment's now on Friday at four fifteen, that's quarter past four.

N Phone call number 3.

W Hello, Mr Watts. You can have an appointment next Tuesday at ten to twelve. All right? Great. So, that's eleven fifty on Tuesday 20 April.

N Phone call number 4.

W I'm sorry, Mr Thomas. I'm afraid the only appointment I have is at a quarter to nine.

N Phone call number 5.

W Hello, Mrs Dobson. I'm sorry but we can't fit you in at 8:30 – we can only do 9:30.

Track 4: Unit 1, Ex. 4: Making appointments

N Phone call number 1.

W Good morning, Epping health centre. Can I help you?

Mrs T Hello. My name's Mrs Taylor, I'd like to make an appointment, please.

W Certainly, is there any particular day or time you would prefer?

Mrs T Yes, is Thursday OK? In the morning?

W We can do Thursday at eight forty if that's OK?

Mrs T That's great, thanks.

W OK, Mrs Taylor, see you on Thursday.

N Phone call number 2.

W Good morning, Epping health centre. Can I help you?

Mr H Yes, Mr Hall here, I'd like to make an appointment, please.

W Certainly, Mr Hall, is there any particular day or time you would prefer?

Mr H Yes, Thursday, late morning, please.

W We can do Thursday at ten past eleven if that's OK?

Mr H That's great, thanks.

W OK, Mr Hall, see you on Thursday.

N Phone call number 3.

W Good morning, Epping health centre. Can I help you?

Mrs M Hi, it's Sandra Marsh. Can I make an appointment, please?

W Certainly, is there any particular day or time you would prefer, Mrs Marsh?

Mrs M Yes, I can do Thursday afternoon. Is that OK?

W Let's see. We can do ten to two in the afternoon?

Mrs M That's great, thanks.

W OK, Mrs Marsh, see you on Thursday.

N Phone call number 4.

W Good afternoon, Epping health centre. Can I help you?

Mrs H Good afternoon, I'd like to make an appointment, please.

W Certainly, is there any particular day or time you would prefer?

Mrs H Yes, is Thursday afternoon OK?

W I'm afraid we're very busy in the afternoon. Can you do half past eleven?

Mrs H Err, OK. That's fine.

W Good. Can I have your name, please?

Mrs H Oh yes, it's Hiley, Susan Hiley. That's H-I-L-E-Y.

W Thanks, Mrs Hiley. See you on Thursday.

Track 5: Unit 1, Ex. 7: Spelling names

N Name number 1.

M Could I have your name, please?

Mrs G Yes, it's Gawlinski. That's G-A-W-L-I-N-S-K-I.

M Thank you, Mrs Gawlinski. And could I have your ...

N Name number 2.

Mr T Good morning. My name is Tuncay. I have an appointment for 10.30.

W Could you spell that please, Mr Tuncay?

Mr T It's T-U-N-C-A-Y.

W Ah, yes. Here you are. Please take a seat, Mr Tuncay.

N Name number 3.

M Could you please spell your name, Mr Kuznetsov?

Mr K Yes, it's K-U-Z-N-E-T-S-O-V.

M That's great. Thank you, Mr Kuznetsov.

N Name number 4.

W How do you spell your name, Mr Yildirim?

Mr Y It's Y-I-L-D-I-R-I-M.

W Right. Thank you, Mr Yildirim.

N Name number 5.

W So, that's Wysocki spelt W-I-Y-S-O ...

Mrs W No, it's spelt W-Y-S-O-C-K-I.

W Oh, I am sorry. Thank you, Mrs Wysocki.

N Name number 6.

M I'm sorry but can you tell me how to spell your name please, Mrs Leigh?

Mrs L Sure. It's L-E-I-G-H.

M Thank you very much, Mrs Leigh.

Mrs L You're welcome.

Track 6: Unit 2, Ex. 1: The practice

N The receptionist makes appointments and answers the phone. The GP diagnoses general health problems. The nurse assists the doctor. The radiologist takes X-rays. The paediatrician specializes in treating children. The physiotherapist helps with joints and movement. The gynaecologist does check-ups for women.

Track 7: Unit 2, Ex. 10: Giving directions

W Mr Singh? Mr Singh? Ah, hello. Dr Alexander can see you now. It's treatment room 2. Go through the doors here and it's the room in front of you.

M Here's the key to the patients' toilets, Mrs Watson. Just go through the doors here and turn left. Go down the corridor and then turn left again and the toilets are on your right.

W Mrs Anderson. Will you go to treatment room 3, please? That's through the doors here and then turn left. Go down the corridor and then it's the third door on your right. It's right at the end of the corridor.

M Hello. Are you from Harlan Medical Supply Company? Can you show me your ID card, please? Thank you. Let me see the delivery note, please. Ah, yes. Six boxes with supplies for the laboratory. Could you take them to the lab, please? The nurse there will check everything and sign the delivery note. Go through the doors here and turn left. Go along the corridor and then left again and it's the third door on your right. Thank you.

W Hello, Mrs Compton from Fife Pharmaceutical Company? Can I see your ID card, please? That's fine, thanks. Dr Bradley is waiting for you in the office. Go through the doors here and then turn left. Go along the corridor and turn left again. It's the room at the end of the corridor.

M Mr Samuels? Please go to the X-ray room, Mr Samuels. That's through the doors here and then turn left. Go down the corridor and turn left. The X-ray room is the first room on your left.

Track 8: Unit 2, Extra Material Ex. 2: Medical history

Kerstin OK, so now I have some more questions for you. Are you having any kind of medical treatment at the moment?

W No, I'm not.

Kerstin Have you ever had an allergic reaction to any kind of treatment before? You know, to drugs, injections or an anaesthetic, for example.

W No, I haven't.

Kerstin Are you taking medication at the moment? If so, what?

W Err, no I'm not. No.

Kerstin Are you pregnant?

W Yes, I am. I'm three months pregnant.

Kerstin OK, so that's three months pregnant. And the next question ... Are you HIV positive?

W No. I'm not.

Kerstin And when did you last see a doctor?

W I haven't been to see a doctor for about a year.

Kerstin And do you have any health problems at the moment?

W No, I don't.

Kerstin OK. Do you have hepatitis B?

W No, I haven't.

Kerstin OK, and finally, do you get anxious when receiving medical treatment?

W Well, I do get a bit nervous about injections, yes.

Track 9: Unit 3, Ex. 5: Seeing the nurse

Sandra Hello, good morning Mr Jarvis. My name's Sandra Waterman. How are you today?

Ron   Very well, thanks.

Sandra   Is this your first visit to our practice?

Ron   Yes, it is. I moved to the town three months ago.

Sandra   Oh really? And where did you live before?

Ron   In a small village called Shepton, about 6 miles away.

Sandra   Oh, I know Shepton very well. Now can you hold this tray for me under your ear? That's great, thanks. And who was your GP there?

Ron   I went to Doctor Wheeler at the Maltings Health Centre.

Sandra   Oh yes, Dr Wheeler's very nice. I lived in Shepton for five years, but I didn't work at the Maltings.

Ron   Where did you work?

Sandra   I worked here. Now I'm going to start syringing your ear. Tell me if it hurts at all, OK? Right here we go. I began working here twenty years ago.

Ron   That's a long time! Did you always want to be a nurse?

Sandra   Yes, I think so. I knew I wanted to be a nurse when I was still at school. This was the first job I applied for when I left school. Is this comfortable for you? It isn't painful at all?

Ron   No, it's fine. I think I can hear better already!

Track 10: Unit 3, Ex. 7: The nose, mouth and throat

W   Right, so that's the ear finished. Now the next part of what we call ENT – or ear, nose and throat – is of course the nose, together with the mouth and the throat. So, if you look in your books at page 21, you can see a diagram of the nose, mouth and throat. Let's begin with the nose. First of all you have the nasal passage at the start of the nose. This is the most important passage for taking air into the body. As air goes through the nasal passage, it passes over the olfactory nerves and these send information about smell to the brain. The air then goes down into the back of the mouth, into the throat and then into the trachea – or windpipe, which carries the air to the lungs. Now if we look at the mouth, we can see the teeth and the lips at the front and then in the middle of the mouth we can see the palate, which is the roof of the mouth, and the tongue, which is of course, the major organ of taste. But remember, smell is also an important part of the way we taste things. Anyway, when we eat or drink, the food goes from the mouth into the back of our throats and when we swallow, it goes into our gullet – or oesophagus –, which is the tube that carries food into the stomach.

Track 11: Unit 3, Ex. 11: What seems to be the problem?

Nurse   Mr Carr. You and your son, Stephen, can see Dr Scott now.

Doctor   Hello, Mr Carr. Hello, Stephen. Now then. What's the problem?

Mr C   Hello, Dr Scott. My son Stephen says his ear hurts. He didn't sleep at all last night and I think he has got a temperature.

Doctor   Well, let's take a look. Stephen, I'd like you to …

Nurse   Mrs Taylor? You can go in now. Dr Scott is ready for you.

Doctor   Good afternoon, Mrs Taylor. You don't look very well today.

Mrs T   I feel terrible, Dr Scott. I keep sneezing, my nose is blocked, but keeps running and I also keep coughing a lot. I don't really feel tired, I just want my nose to stop running.

Doctor   I'd like you to open your mouth and say …

Nurse   Mr Tuncay? Please go in. Dr Scott will see you now.

Doctor   Please sit down, Mr Tuncay.

Mr T   Thank you, Dr Scott. I really don't feel very well.

Doctor   Can you describe your symptoms?

Mr T   Yes, I think I have a temperature. I feel really tired and my arms and shoulders ache. And my nose keeps running, and I have a sore throat.

Doctor   Do you cough at all?

Mr T   Yes, quite often.

Doctor   I see. Please take off your shirt, Mr Tuncay. I'd like to …

Nurse   You can go in now, Mrs Anderson.

Doctor   Hello, Mrs Anderson. Please sit down and tell me what's wrong.

Mrs A   Hello, Dr Scott. I feel terrible. My stomach is really painful and I keep vomiting and I have a fever. I keep feeling hot and then cold.

Doctor   Do you have diarrhoea, as well?

Mrs A   Yes, I do.

Doctor   When did all this start, Mrs Anderson?

Mrs A   Well, I first noticed that I had a temperature last …

Nurse   Hello, Mrs Morris. You and your daughter can go in now.

Doctor   Hello, Mrs Morris. And who is this pretty little girl?

Mrs M   This is Lucy, Dr Scott. Say hello to Dr Scott, Lucy.
Sorry, she's very shy.

Doctor   Never mind. Could you describe your daughter's symptoms, Mrs Morris?

Mrs M   Yes, Lucy says she has a headache and doesn't feel well. I took her temperature and I think she has a fever. She also has a rash of small red spots on her chest. Her nose keeps running and she has a bit of a cough, as well.

Doctor   OK, Mrs Morris, I'd like you to bring Lucy over here. I'd like to take a look at that rash first. And then I'd like to …

Track 12: Unit 3, Ex. 13: Examining the patient

Nurse   Mr Carter. The doctor can see you now.

Andrew   Oh, great.

Nurse   It's treatment room three. The one on the right.

Andrew   OK. Thanks.

Dr Grant   Good morning, Mr Carter. What's the problem?

Andrew   I've cut my arm, doctor.

Dr Grant   OK. Then let's take a look at it. Could you roll up your sleeve, please?

Andrew   Sure.

Dr Grant   That's better. Hmm. When did this happen?

Andrew   This morning. I was trying to take the chain off my bike. I was using a screwdriver and it slipped. I cleaned the cut and put a bandage on it.

Dr Grant   Well, you did the right thing. It's a long cut, but it isn't very deep. And it's very clean and should heal quickly. Don't worry, it will only need two or three stitches. Have you had a tetanus injection recently?

Andrew   I had one five or six years ago, but I can't remember when exactly.

Dr Grant   Well, you'll need a tetanus injection.

Andrew   OK.

Dr Grant   But first I'll clean and disinfect the cut before I start with the stitches. Just hold out your arm, Mr Carter and …

Track 13: Unit 4, Ex. 4: Stitching a wound

Dr Grant   So, Mr Carter, this is going to sting.

Patient   Ooo!

Dr Grant   I'm just cleaning the wound before I start stitching. Good. And now the hypodermic, please Caroline. This is just a local anaesthetic, Mr Carter, so you won't feel the stitches.

Patient   OK, thanks.

Dr Grant   It'll take a minute or two for the anaesthetic to take effect. I'll be back in a minute or two, Mr Carter. Please get everything ready for the stitches, Caroline.

Nurse   Yes, doctor.

Nurse   Don't worry, Mr Carter. You'll hardly feel a thing. Have you lived here long?

Patient   No, only a year or two. I moved here after my wife died. I wanted to be near my son and his family.

Nurse   That's good – that you're near your family, I mean. Oh, here comes Dr Grant.

Dr Grant   The anaesthetic should be ready now, so we can start. Have you got everything ready, Caroline?

Nurse   Yes, Dr Grant. Here's the needle with thread and a needle holder.

Dr Grant   Thank you. Now, Mr Carter. If you wish, you can look in the other direction while I stitch the cut.

Patient   No, I'm fine, thanks. I can feel it, but it doesn't hurt.

Dr Grant   Good. I'm almost finished. There we are. Now I just have to tie off the stitches. That's it. Caroline will put a dressing on that, Mr Carter. Come back in ten days and we'll take the stitches out.

Patient   That's great. Thanks very much, doctor.

Nurse   OK, Mr Carter. Hold out your arm and I'll …

Track 14: Unit 4, Ex. 6: Taking blood

Mary   Good morning. I'm Mary Smith and I have an appointment for a blood test and an immunization against hepatitis A.

Kerstin   Oh yes. Good morning, Mrs Smith. I'll take you straight to the treatment room. It's along here on the left. Here we are. Please wait here and I'll tell Dr Müller that you are here and waiting for your immunization.

Mary   OK, thanks.

Kerstin   Here I am again, Mrs Smith. I can take the blood sample while we're waiting for Dr Müller. Could you take off your jacket and roll up your sleeve, please?

Mary   Is that high enough?

Kerstin   That's fine. Now, I'm just putting on a tourniquet before I take the sample. Does that feel OK? Not too tight?

Mary   No, that's fine.

Kerstin   Good. And now the needle. This might hurt a little bit – but not much. There we are. That's it. Now I'll take the blood samples. Best to look away, Mrs Smith. Lots of people don't like the sight of blood. There – I'm finished. That didn't take long, did it? Now I can take off the tourniquet, take out the needle and we're done.

Mary   Great. I'm glad that's over!

Kerstin   Yes, the worst is over. Could you just hold this cottonwool swab on your arm for a minute or two, please?

Mary   Sure.

Kerstin   Right. I'll put a plaster on and then we're done. Please wait here, Mrs Smith. Dr Müller will be with you in a minute or two for the immunization. OK?

Mary   Yes, thank you.

N Julie Peters goes to a pharmacy in Hamburg to get a prescription filled for a hepatitis A injection. Katrin Scholl works at the pharmacy.

Katrin Guten Tag. Kann ich Ihnen helfen?

Julie Oh, I'm sorry, but I don't speak German. Can you help me?

Katrin Yes, I hope so. How can I help you?

Julie I have this prescription from my doctor. It's for a hepatitis A injection.

Katrin Oh, yes. We've got that. Just a moment. ... Ah, yes, here it is.

Julie I've also got a bad cough. Can you give me something for it, please?

Katrin Is it a chesty cough?

Julie No, it's a dry cough in my throat.

Katrin Do you have any other symptoms?

Julie Yes, I often get a headache, too. I think I'm coming down with a cold.

Katrin Well, it could just be a cold. But you might be getting the flu. I hope it isn't the flu.

Julie Why?

Katrin Because if it really is the flu, then you won't be able to have the hepatitis injection. You must talk to your doctor. So, here's the cough mixture for your throat and some paracetamol for your headache.

Julie Err ... Is this the dosage here on the packet? What does it say?

Katrin You can take one or two paracetamol tablets three or four times a day. But don't take more than eight in one day.

Julie OK. And the cough medicine?

Katrin It says: one or two teaspoonfuls every four hours.

Julie Thank you very much. You've been a great help. How much is that altogether?

Katrin That's 95 euros for the hepatitis A vaccine, 2 euros 50 for the paracetamol and 15 euros for the cough mixture. So, that's 112 euros 50 altogether, please.

Julie Can I pay by card?

Katrin No problem. Would you like a bag?

Julie No, thanks, I've got ...

Sarila Hello, Paul. This is Sarila at Dr Fischer's practice.

Paul Hello, Sarila. What can I do for you?

Sarila My last order has been delivered. I've got the delivery note here and I'm afraid there are several mistakes.

Paul Oh, are some things missing?

Sarila Well, all the things in the delivery note are in the shipment, but ...

Paul So nothing is missing?

Sarila Paul, the delivery note is wrong. This isn't what I ordered.

Paul Hold on, I'm just calling up your last order.

Sarila I've got it here in front of me. I'll read it to you. First of all, I wanted 10 one-litre bottles of saline infusion.

Paul Oh, yes. And we've delivered 20 half-litre bottles. I'm sorry about that.

Sarila Look, Paul. I can live with that. After all, it's the same amount. But the other mistakes are more serious.

Paul I think I know what the problem is. We've had a few minor problems with our computer software.

Sarila A few minor problems? Paul, I only ordered 2 infusion pumps – not 20! And I wanted 15 doses of tetanus vaccine. You've sent us 150! That's far too much.

Paul Oh, my goodness.

Sarila And I ordered 40 boxes of gauze bandages.

Paul And we have only sent four. Is anything at all correct?

Sarila Yes, the examination gloves and the disposable syringes are correct. You have sent the correct amount for those.

Paul Well, that's something. What's next?

Sarila General disinfectant. You've delivered one bottle, but I ordered ten. And I wanted 30 tins of antiseptic ointment, not three. That will only last us till the end of the week.

Paul Sarila, I'm very sorry about this. I'll send you the missing items express and you'll have them tomorrow morning. OK? We'll also pick up the things you don't need.

Sarila OK, fair enough – as long as everything arrives sometime tomorrow.

Paul Everything will be there before 5 p.m., I promise. And I'm really very sorry about the mix-up. It won't happen again.

Nurse Do you want to make another appointment, Mr Thompson?

Mr T Not at the moment, thanks. But I don't know this town very well. Is there a pharmacy near here where I can fill my prescription?

Nurse The nearest pharmacy is about ten minutes from here on foot, but it's only a minute or two by car.

Mr T I'll walk there. The exercise will do me good. Can you tell me how to get there?

Nurse Yes, and I'll draw a sketch for you. When you leave the practice turn right and walk to the next crossroads. There's a big health centre on the corner. Cross the road using the pedestrian subway. You'll come to a crossroads. Cross over Bismarckstraße and go straight ahead until you reach the corner.

The pharmacy is then opposite you on the other side of the road.

Mr T That's very helpful. Thanks.

Track 18: Unit 5, Ex. 10: Another medical practice

Patient Can you tell me how to get to the bus station from here, please?

Nurse Yes, certainly. Do you want to walk or take the bus?

Patient I'd prefer to walk if it isn't too far.

Nurse It'll take you about twenty minutes on foot.

Patient That's fine. I've got plenty of time.

Nurse OK. When you leave here, cross the road to the pharmacy on the corner.

Patient Oh, yes. I saw it when I came in.

Nurse OK. So then you turn left at the corner. Walk along Schillerstraße until you reach the fourth crossroads. You'll see the bus station on your left. It's a big place. There's a pedestrian subway at the crossroads. It will take you straight to the bus station.

Patient Well, that sounds easy enough. Thanks for your help.

Nurse You're welcome. Have a nice day. Bye.

Patient Bye.

Track 19: Unit 6, Ex. 1: Different people have different needs

Mike I'm Mike Sheffield and this is my daughter, Shelley. She's here for a smallpox vaccination. I've told her that it won't hurt, but she's still anxious. A doctor's practice is a scary place for a young kid.

Susan My name is Susan Farrows. I'm 16 and I'm here for a pelvic examination. I've never had a pelvic examination before and I'm feeling a bit nervous.

Rachel I'm Rachel Monahan. I really just want to renew my prescription medication. Normally I just phone in and the doctor sends it to me by post, but this time the doctor wants to take some blood and urine samples first. My husband has taken a day off work so that he can drive me here and then pick me up later and take me home.

Li My name is Yao Li and I'm from Canton. I'm a student here. I was at the beach with some friends and I cut my foot on a broken bottle. It isn't a serious cut, but I think I should have a tetanus injection.

Barney I'm Barney Redford. I've got an awful pain in my back. I haven't been here for a couple of years. I don't like going to the doctor's. You have to sit in a waiting room with people coughing and spreading their germs. You never know what diseases they might have.

Track 20: Unit 6, Ex. 9: Dealing with anxious patients

Nurse Doctor, that was great the way you dealt with that nervous patient.

Doctor Thank you. Do you know, I've been a doctor now for nearly 30 years and the patients still have the same old fears as when I started!

Nurse How do you mean?

Doctor Well, medicine has changed so much in the last 30 years but people still fear the same things. Take injections, for example, a lot of people still get really nervous about getting injections – everyone remembers how painful they were as a kid – but now we use smaller needles and make sure that giving an injection or taking blood is as comfortable and painless as possible.

Nurse I remember my doctor when I was a kid. He was really scary!

Doctor I know. And 30 years ago doctors weren't expected to spend so much time with their patients. We're all told now that we should spend more time talking to our patients and listening to them, and we should always explain the risks and the benefits of each treatment. I suppose if it means patients don't feel so helpless and anxious, then it's a good idea.

Nurse But not all doctors are friendly like you, Dr Graham.

Doctor Well, I try, but like many doctors I don't really have much more time for my patients now than doctors had thirty years ago. And I guess some doctors today think that progress in diagnosis and medication means that they don't have to talk to their patients! But the patient has got to trust you or they shouldn't start the treatment. And the instruments! In the old days, they used to be really big and scary!

Nurse But instruments nowadays are much smaller. Many instruments are now digital and less invasive.

Doctor That's right. And they worry that we're too busy and don't have time to do our job properly – so we need to make a relaxed atmosphere and not look rushed.

Nurse And I bet they didn't have TVs in the waiting room when you started!

Doctor That's true! Or soft music playing in the surgery … I know a doctor who burns aromatherapy candles in his office …

Nurse No! I even read about one who gave foot spas and massages in his surgery!

Doctor I think that's going a bit far! I'm sure the patients all love these things, but I don't think they really relieve anxiety any better than simply listening to the patient and explaining what you're doing!

Susan   Er, hello? I've got an appointment for 10.30.

Meike   Ah, yes. Here we are, Miss Farrows. It's Susan, isn't it?

Susan   Yes, that's right.

Meike   And you're here for a pelvic exam. Is this your first one?

Susan   Er, yes, it is.

Meike   OK. Please follow me. I'll take you to a treatment room. There's nothing to worry about. It won't hurt at all. Here we are. Now, before the doctor comes, I need to measure your blood pressure. Please take your jacket off, Susan, and roll up the sleeve of your right arm. That's it, thank you. OK. Your blood pressure is a little high today. Are you nervous, Susan?

Susan   A bit, yes.

Meike   There's nothing to be nervous about, it's just a routine check-up. Do you know what happens in the exam?

Susan   Not really, no. That's why I'm a bit nervous.

Meike   It's OK, that's normal the first time. Well, when you see the doctor he'll ask you some routine questions first. Then he'll explain everything to you and make sure you feel completely comfortable.

Susan   Great. Will he examine my breasts, too?

Meike   Yes, he'll ask you to undress and he'll examine your breasts while you stand in front of him. He'll show you how to do a self exam, too. Look, would you like me to be present?

Susan   No, it's OK. I think I'll be all right.

Meike   You will be, don't worry.

Susan   What happens after that?

Meike   Then you lie down on the exam table. He has to take what we call a smear test – which is taking some cells from your cervix using a tiny wooden stick and a special brush. Don't worry, it's just routine, but it means we can send the cells for testing and make sure everything is absolutely as it should be.

Susan   Is that everything?

Meike   Almost. Last of all, the doctor does a quick internal examination to make sure all your internal organs are just as they should be. It won't hurt, but if you do feel any discomfort, tell the doctor right away. The doctor will explain in more detail exactly what he's going to do at each step of the examination. He's very gentle and really friendly, you know. Just sit down and relax, Susan. He'll be with you in a minute or two. OK?

Susan   OK. Thanks.

Joyce   Good afternoon everyone. My name is Joyce Reynolds and I'm here today to talk to you about the relationship between a patient and a carer. The success of everything we do as carers relies on trust and human understanding. Our patients' situation means that they need other people to do some of the basic and personal tasks for them. However, they still have the same human dignity as everyone else. So we must always, therefore, show warmth, understanding and respect. This means always remembering a few simple, but very important, points.

Firstly, as we all know, patients often get angry and frustrated. It's essential to keep calm, not react and not take it personally. Try to find out why the patient is angry. The patient might not even know that he or she is ill-tempered and even if they do, they might not know why. They are probably lonely or worried rather than angry with you.

Secondly, by doing too much for a patient you can create a feeling of helplessness and weakness. Even worse, the patient can become lazy and simply expect you to do everything, which will make your job harder and reduce their self-respect. So, remember to let the patients do things for themselves – it will make your life easier and increase their self-esteem.

Next, it's important to remember the job is all about people. But rushing around doing jobs for the patient can mean that there is little or no time to actually be with the patient. If the patient thinks you are too busy, he or she might not even try to talk to you. And remember: listening is one of the most important things a carer does.

Honesty is the next point. If the patient is angry because of something you have done, tell the truth, apologize and try to put things right. Don't make the same mistake again. Always tell the truth. If you have forgotten something, say so. Without honesty there can be no trust.

And finally, don't forget to take care of yourself, as well. As a carer, you get tired and frustrated. Take time off to relax and do things you enjoy. Make sure that there's someone you can talk to about the difficulties of the job. You could talk to your manager, but sometimes it is better to talk to someone outside of work.

N First caller.

Hotline Good morning, NHS Nutrition Hotline. How can I help you?

Caller 1 Oh, good morning. Could you give me some information about a healthy diet during pregnancy, please?

Hotline Certainly. One of the best things I can recommend for pregnant women is folic acid. You find it in fruit and vegetables such as cabbage, broccoli and spinach. It's also in high-fibre food such as bread and cereals.

Caller 1 What about vitamins? Should I take extra vitamins?

Hotline Well, some are more useful than others. Vitamin C and D, for example, are very good for you, but too much vitamin A or B can be dangerous. You should really discuss this with your doctor.

Caller 1 Oh, I see. Umm, I have another question. Is it really true that you can't drink any alcohol while you're pregnant?

Hotline Yes, you really shouldn't. Alcohol can harm the foetus. And don't forget: no smoking either.

Caller 1 It's OK, I'm not a smoker, anyway. Oh, one other thing …

N Second caller.

Hotline Good morning, NHS Nutrition Hotline. How can I help you?

Caller 2 Hello. I have a question about the labels on some products. When I read them, I see there are lots of different types of oils and fats. Could you tell me what the difference is between them and which ones are healthier than others?

Hotline Well, first, there are vegetable oils, like olive oil and rapeseed oil, for example. And then there are animal fats.

Caller 2 By animal fats, you mean butter, right?

Hotline Yes, butter and fat found in other dairy products, like milk or yoghurt, but also fat from meat like beef, pork, chicken, …

Caller 2 I see.

Hotline Some vegetable oils, like olive oil or rapeseed oil – in the USA this is called 'canola oil' – are a lot healthier for you than animal fats. Too much animal fat in your diet can cause high blood pressure and heart problems because they increase the cholesterol levels in the blood.

Caller 2 What are the most dangerous types of fats?

Hotline Well, beef fat is more harmful than fats found in chicken and fish. And some vegetable oils, like coconut oil or palm oil, are just as bad. They're all high in something called saturated fats. Doctors say we should limit the amount of saturated fats in our diets.

Caller 2 Err, what do you mean by the word 'saturated'?

Hotline Well, all the fat we eat …

N Third caller.

Hotline Good morning, NHS Nutrition Hotline. How can I help you?

Caller 3 Good morning. I'm calling about baby food products.

Hotline OK. Any products in particular?

Caller 3 Yes, my baby daughter really likes drinking sweet tea, but a friend of mine said that it isn't good for her. Is that true?

Hotline Well, sweet tea contains a lot of sugar and too much sugar is very bad for your baby's teeth. So, yes, unsweetened teas are better for her.

Caller 3 But what if she doesn't like them? I think my daughter has a bit of a sweet tooth, so she might not like unsweetened tea.

Hotline Well, some fruit teas don't need any sugar because they are naturally sweet. In fact, some fruit teas are naturally sweeter than some of the teas sweetened with sugar. They are some of the most popular baby products. They're very good. But you can also buy some baby drinks that taste sweet but don't have any sugar in them. Maybe you can try the unsweetened fruit teas first and if your daughter really doesn't like them, then you could try the others.

Caller 3 OK, I'll do that. Thanks for your help. Bye.

MA So, you've seen the doctor. Was it all OK?

Magda Yes, he told me to speak to you about things I can do every day to help.

MA Did he say if you will need tablets or insulin injections?

Magda He's prescribed some tablets, but I don't need injections.

MA That's good news. One of the most important things is to take day-to-day control of your diabetes yourself and make the right changes to your lifestyle.

Magda Do you mean don't eat chocolate and things like that?

MA No, chocolate is actually OK – if it's part of a healthy diet. It's really simple things like a healthy diet, losing a bit of weight and more physical activity.

Magda Is that all?

MA That and learning about self-care. I'll give you some information on diet and how you can learn to monitor your own blood glucose levels. There are some really simple things you can do like checking your feet for signs of high blood glucose levels.

Magda My feet?

MA I know! It sounds crazy but it's true. It's all in the information here. You'll need to work with your diabetes care team – that's us. Talk regularly with us and learn when to ask for help if you're ill or get a chest infection, for example. We'll make some regular appointments and it's really important that you keep them so that the team knows you're making the right changes to your daily lifestyle and your diabetes is under control. Type 2 diabetes is progressive – so if you don't control it, it can get worse and cause damage to your nerves, heart and arteries.

Track 25: Unit 8, Ex. 1: Seeing the doctor

Dr Müller Ah, Ms Michaels. Please, come in. What can I do for you?

Julia Well, I haven't been feeling well for a while now and it's hard to explain, but I just don't have any energy any more, and I feel weak – sort of like I have the flu. And I also have a strange feeling in my legs – it's like pins and needles or when your leg goes to sleep when you sit on it for a while or something like that. It's kind of a weird feeling.

Dr Müller I see. Well, I'm just going to ask you some questions to find out more about your symptoms.

Julia Well, you see doctor, I went on the Internet and looked up my symptoms and started reading about MS, which made me depressed, so I thought I'd better come and talk to someone.

Dr Müller Well, you're right to come to see me, but those symptoms could mean a lot of things, Ms Michaels. You shouldn't assume the worst, you know. Have you had any other symptoms such as any problems with your vision at all?

Julia No, I haven't. But what about the strange tingling in my legs?

Dr Müller Sensations like that can be perfectly normal – or caused by many things. Are you having bladder or bowel difficulties?

Julia Not really, no.

Dr Müller Then I wouldn't worry too much about having no energy. Have you had any difficulties with coordination or balance at all?

Julia Yeah, I have actually. The other day I suddenly felt very dizzy and had to sit down. I thought maybe I just stood up too quickly or something.

Dr Müller Hmm. Has it happened again since then?

Julia Not really, no. But the pins and needles feeling is still there. And I feel really down at the moment.

Dr Müller Hmm. Well, Ms Michaels, what we're going to do today is take a blood sample and then send it off for analysis. But don't get all worried about MS.

Julia When will I get the results?

Dr Müller It's normally 3-4 days. Reception will give you another appointment for when the results come back. But don't worry about it. Blood tests are very routine. It's just to be on the safe side and find out if there's an infection of some kind. And I'd also like to do a complete physical examination, if that's all right.

Julia OK. Sure.

Dr Müller So, if you'd like to remove your jacket and roll up your sleeve. I'm just going to take a blood sample.

Julia Are you going to use a needle?

Dr Müller Yes, but don't worry, this isn't going to hurt at all and it's all …

Track 26: Unit 8, Ex. 6: An MRI scan

Heike Hello Ms Michaels. My name's Heike and I'm going to look after you today.

Julia Hi. Nice to meet you.

Heike Is this the first time you've had a scan?

Julia Yes, it is. And I'm a little nervous.

Heike No need to worry. The scanner is like a big camera and we're going to take some pictures of you. It's all very safe. Now, have you filled in the questionnaire?

Julia Err, yes. Here it is.

Heike Great. Thanks. OK, so this all looks good. So you have nothing metal in you at all? That's good! Now, I'm going to have to ask you to undress and put this gown on. And you need to take off everything that is metal, like your watch or any jewellery. And could you please take off your bra as it has metal clasps – we can't put anything metal in the scanner, you see.

Julia Oh, OK.

Heike That's great. Here let me help you with the gown. OK, now could you please lie back on the table? In a minute I'm going to move the table into the scanner and we can start scanning. The scanner can be a bit noisy, so put these earplugs in. That's it. And can I just put your head in between these pads here? That's perfect. And it can be a bit cold, so I'm just going to put a blanket over you. OK? Great. Now when the machine starts, it will make a loud banging noise for a minute or so and then go quiet for a few seconds, and then start again. The whole thing should last about 45 minutes. Are you comfortable?

Julia Yes, thanks.

Heike Good. Now I'm going to leave the room but don't worry, I'm going to keep talking to you and telling you what's happening. Right, let's get started!

Track 27: Unit 8, Ex. 12: How MS progresses

N In its early stages, Multiple Sclerosis can be very hard to diagnose. In fact, a definite diagnosis is often only possible by ruling out other diseases – unless there are regular separate attacks or a steady decline over a period of at least six months. Once the disease has been diagnosed, doctors will identify which of the four subtypes of MS the patient's symptoms are showing. This will help the doctor predict the future course of the disease.

The first of these subtypes is what we call Relapsing-remitting MS. This is the form of the disease that affects 90% of patients in the early stages and describes separate attacks – or relapses – followed by quiet periods of remission that can last months or even years.

Most people who suffer Relapsing-remitting MS in the early stages, then go on to have more frequent attacks until the symptoms just start growing steadily worse without the quiet periods in between. This is the most common form of MS and is called Second-ary-progressive MS.

Next we have what's called Primary-pro-gressive MS, when the symptoms just get steadily worse right from the very early stages of the disease. This is pretty uncom-mon with only about 10% of sufferers having Primary-progressive MS.

And finally we have Progressive-relapsing MS, the least common form of all, when the symptoms get steadily worse but the patient also suffers bad attacks of the disease at regular intervals.

Track 28: Unit 9, Ex. 2: Symptoms of eating disorders

W Eating disorders are a growing problem for young people today. With glossy magazines full of size zero, it's easy to see why teenagers are suffering from low self-esteem and problems with accepting their weight. With me today is Dr Sanjay Sohail, who is an expert on eating disorders. Good morning, Dr Sohail.

Dr S Good morning.

W First of all, what are the most common eating disorders?

Dr S Well, there are three main disorders: anorexia, bulimia and overeating.

W And how are they different?

Dr S Basically, anorexia is when someone doesn't eat enough to keep their body weight. Overeating is when someone eats far more than they need to keep their body weight, and bulimia is overeating followed by purging.

W What do you mean by 'purging'?

Dr S Purging is when someone overeats and then makes themselves vomit to bring all the food back up in order to control their body weight.

W Now, parents often don't see the symptoms soon enough. So maybe you could tell us how to spot these illnesses.

Dr S Well, people who suffer from anorexia and bulimia starve their body of the food and energy it needs, which can lead to serious weight loss. It can also lead to poor circulation, low blood pressure, feeling cold, headaches, and no energy or enthusiasm. Because the body also doesn't get the vitamins it needs, hair loss is common as is the growth of facial hair. Malnutrition also leads to dental problems. Bulimics eat large amounts of food because they are de-pressed, then they purge by either vomiting it back up or using a strong laxative.

W It all sounds horrible! And what about overeating? We hear a lot about teenage obesity nowadays.

Dr S Being overweight is the easiest symptom to see. Sufferers often have high blood pressure and a fast or irregular heart rate. All these illnesses can lead to depression, too, of course.

W And what can parents do when they see these symptoms?

Dr S I think it's very important that they don't try to deal with it themselves. They should talk to their family doctor and …

Track 29: Unit 9, Ex. 6: A growing weight problem

Presenter Hello, and welcome back. Now, I don't know about you but it seems to me that kids nowa-days are getting bigger and bigger. There's lots of talk about teenagers eating junk food and playing video games all day, but I wonder, are kids really getting bigger? And if so, why? So, with me in the studio is Dr Sherry Bonheim from the National Obesity Forum. So, Sherry, are kids getting bigger?

Expert Yes, they are. A new study shows that

amongst 10 to 17-year-olds, about 30 per cent of kids are now overweight or obese. In 49 US states, one in five people are now obese.

Presenter One in five! That's incredible. But how overweight is 'obese'?

Expert People with a BMI of over 30 are …

Presenter BM what?

Expert BMI. Body mass index. It's your weight in kilograms divided by the square of your height in metres. A healthy BMI is between 18 and 25, anything over 30 is obese.

Presenter But why are so many people overweight?

Expert Well, there are many reasons. There has been a lot of research and it seems kids today do far less physical activity than before. And kids are eating a lot more calories, too.

Presenter People are eating more …

Expert Yes, and less healthy food – more fast food and high-calorie foods.

Presenter And what else does research tell us?

Expert It also tells us that kids hang out with other kids of the same weight and copy each other's eating habits.

Presenter So fat friends can make you overweight!

Expert Yes, so it seems …

Presenter But what about parents? Surely they play a part in this?

Expert They do. If dad's overweight, then he's less likely to go out and play soccer with the kids, so they join him on the couch and watch TV together.

Presenter And how big a problem is all this?

Expert Well, obesity increases the risk of type 2 diabetes and there are now over 20 million Americans with diabetes. Health care spending on obesity rose by 37 per cent between 1996 and 2008 and now costs the US over 150 billion dollars a year.

Presenter Now, that's what I call a big problem! But what can we do about …

Track 30: Unit 10, Ex. 4: Looking for work

N Ulrike, age 24

Ulrike Well, it's a bit harder for me because I'm not actually British. I'm living in England because my husband is British. We moved here two years ago and I've been working in shops and stuff. But I trained as a doctor's assistant in Germany, so I'd like to make use of my training and start a career in the UK. The trouble is, you don't really have a similar qualification in the UK and you don't have doctor's assistants here. When I worked in a small practice in Germany for three years, for example, I did all the reception work and helped the doctor treat patients. No one

does both jobs in the UK. I'll need to learn what software is used here, but I'm sure that won't be a problem.

N Sharon, age 32

Sharon I worked as a general practice nurse for six years before I stopped to have children. Before I stopped, I was a team leader responsible for a team of five nurses. I'd got my RN qualification and was studying for a post-graduate diploma. One of my children is disabled, so I've learnt a lot about caring for the disabled while I've been a full-time mother. I'd like to go back to full-time work now my children are at school.

N Tom, age 17

Tom I'm about to finish school and I really want to find a job, but I haven't really got any qualifications. I'm doing a Saturday job at the moment in an old people's home, which I really enjoy. The old people have lots of really interesting stories about what life was like when they were young. Sometimes they're really funny, as well. I wouldn't mind working with old people as a full-time job if I could find one.

N Kate, age 22

Kate When I left school, I went to college and did a National Vocational Qualification course in Health and Social Care. I worked with old people for a while and really enjoyed it, but I lost my job after about a year. So, I went to a temping agency and did some temporary secretarial jobs for a while. I think I'm good at getting on with people and I'd like to work with the elderly again. What else? Well, I'm good with computers and I think I'm also pretty good at organizing.

Track 31: Unit 10, Ex. 12: Preparing for an interview

Presenter So, next we're going to talk about job interviews. With the help of my next guest, you too can go into a job interview feeling relaxed and confident. So, welcome Sophie McKenzie, from Elite Employment. Hello Sophie.

Sophie Hi.

Presenter So, Sophie. It's the day of the interview. What can you do to make it all less stressful?

Sophie Well, the day of the interview is too late to start thinking about it. You need to do lots of preparation beforehand!

Presenter Oh, right. And what kind of preparation is that?

Sophie Well, for a start, find out everything you can about the company. Can you find information about them on the internet, for example? Can you talk to someone who works there? And always make sure you know where the interview will be. How long will it take you to get there? If you're going by car, what will the traffic be like at that time of day? Never be late for an interview.

Presenter That all sounds very sensible. What else can you do to prepare?

Sophie Find out about the job. Read the advertisement very carefully, several times. If you need to, change your CV to match it the best you can and think carefully about how to explain why you are right for the job. Practise the interview with a friend. Record it and listen to how you sound. Don't forget, practice makes perfect.

Presenter And what about appearances? How important is it to look smart?

Sophie Very important. Always choose clothes that are smart but comfortable. Avoid lots of jewellery or clothes that look sexy. Don't wear new clothes or shoes for the first time as they may be uncomfortable. Once again, plan in advance.

Presenter OK, that's lots of preparation, but what about the big day itself?

Sophie The best preparation starts the evening before your interview. Have a relaxing bath. It will help you to relax and get a good night's sleep. Get up early enough so that you have enough time for a good healthy breakfast and give yourself plenty of time to get to the interview.

Presenter That's great advice. Thank you very much Sophie McKenzie.

Talking about numbers

Cardinal numbers		Ordinal numbers	
0	oh/nought/null (AE) zero		
1	one	1st	first
2	two	2nd	second
3	three	3rd	third
4	four	4th	fourth
5	five	5th	fifth
6	six	6th	sixth
7	seven	7th	seventh
8	eight	8th	eighth
9	nine	9th	ninth
10	ten	10th	tenth
11	eleven	11th	eleventh
12	twelve	12th	twelfth
13	thirteen	13th	thirteenth
14	fourteen	14th	fourteenth
15	fifteen	15th	fifteenth
16	sixteen	16th	sixteenth
17	seventeen	17th	seventeenth
18	eighteen	18th	eighteenth
19	nineteen	19th	nineteenth
20	twenty	20th	twentieth
21	twenty-one	21st	twenty-first
22	twenty-two	22nd	twenty-second
23	twenty-three	23rd	twenty-third
24	twenty-four	24th	twenty-fourth
30	thirty	30th	thirtieth
40	forty	40th	fortieth

Cardinal numbers		Ordinal numbers	
50	fifty	50th	fiftieth
60	sixty	60th	sixtieth
70	seventy	70th	seventieth
80	eighty	80th	eightieth
90	ninety	90th	ninetieth
100	one hundred	100th	one hundredth

In English you say:

101	one hundred **and** one
235	two hundred **and** thirty-five
1,563,765	one million, five hundred **and** sixty-three thousand, seven
1 563 765	hundred **and** sixty-five

You use commas or spaces (and not a point) after the thousands (or millions) in large numbers.

Decimals

In English, you write decimals with a point, not a comma.

0.25	oh/nought point two five (BE) zero point two five (AE)
3.76	three point seven six
55.37	fifty-five point three seven
1.585	one point five eight five

Fractions

¼	a/one quarter
⅓	a/one third
½	a/one half
⅔	two-thirds
¾	three-quarters
⁵⁄₁₆	five sixteenths
1½	one and a half

$1\ m^2$	one **square** metre
$1\ m^3$	one **cubic** metre
5^2	five **squared**
10^4	ten **to the power** of four
+ plus	x times/multiply by
– minus	÷ divide by

Talking about measurements

Taking temperature

The 'normal' body temperature is 37°C (thirty-seven degrees Centigrade/Celsius). That's 98.6°F (ninety-eight point six degrees Fahrenheit).
– He has a temperature of 38°C.
– She's ill in bed with a temperature of 102°F.
– If your temperature goes above 100°F, give me a call.

Measuring blood pressure (BP)

– Your blood pressure's normal. It's 120/80 (one twenty over eighty).
– He's suffering from high blood pressure. Today's reading is 185/100 (one eighty-five over one hundred).

Other measurements and their abbreviations

mg	milligram
g	gram
kg	kilogram
oz	ounce (= 28.35 g)
lb	pound (= 0.454 kg)
st	stone (= 6.356 kg)
ml	millilitre
cl	centilitre
l	litre
tsp	teaspoon
tbl	tablespoon

Conversion tables

Length:

1 inch	=	2.54 cm
1 foot	=	30.48 cm
1 yard	=	91.44 cm
1 mile	=	1.609 km
1 cm	=	0.3937 inches

1 m	=	39.37 inches
1 km	=	0.62137 miles

Area:

1 square inch (in^2)	=	6.45 cm^2
1 square foot (ft^2)	=	0.093 m^2
1 square mile (m^2)	=	2.59 km^2
1 cm^2	=	0.155 square inches
1 m^2	=	10.764 square feet
1 km^2	=	0.3861 square miles

Volume:

1 cubic inch (in^3)	=	16.387 cm^3
1 pint (pt.)	=	0.57 l
1 gallon (gal.)	=	4.546 l
1 US gallon	=	3.785 l
1 cm^3	=	0.061 cubic inch
1 m^3	=	35.315 cubic feet
1 litre (l)	=	1.76 pints
1 litre (l)	=	0.22 gallons

Mass:

1 pound (lb)	=	0.453 kg
1 ton (t)	=	1016 kg
1 kilogram (kg)	=	2.2046 pounds

Temperature:

Degrees Celsius	Degrees Fahrenheit
–17.8°C	= 0°F
–12.2°C	= 10°F
–6.7°C	= 20°F
–1.1°C	= 30°F

You say: –5°C minus five degrees Celsius
–25.5°C minus twenty-five point five degrees Celsius

0°C	= 32°F
4.4°C	= 40°F

10°C	=	50°F
20°C	=	68°F
30°C	=	86°F
40°C	=	104°F
50°C	=	122°F

Absolute zero = –273.15°C

Energy:

1 joule = 0.2388 calories (cal)

Talking about time and dates

Telling the time

7.00	7 o'clock (in the morning)
	seven a.m.
7.05	5 minutes past seven
	seven oh five a.m.
7.15	(a) quarter past seven
	seven fifteen a.m.
7.30	half past seven
	seven thirty a.m.
7.45	(a) quarter to eight
	seven forty-five a.m.
7.57	3 minutes to/before eight
	seven fifty-seven a.m.
12.00	twelve o'clock (noon/midday)
3.00	three o'clock (in the afternoon)
	three p.m.
3.30	half past three
	three thirty p.m.
12.00	twelve o'clock (at night)
	midnight

a.m. = from 0.00 to 12.00 (you say: ay – em)
p.m. = from 12.00 to 0.00 (you say: pee – em)
o'clock is only used for the full hour

Formal:
What time is it, please?
Can you tell me what the time is, please?

Informal:
What's the time?

What's the date today?

you write:	you say:
8 July	It's the eighth of July.
8th August	It's the eighth of August
July 8th	It's July the eighth. (BE)
	It's July eighth. (AE)

Be careful:
8.7.01 means '8 July 2001' in the UK, but
'August 7, 2001' in the USA!

Days of the week

Monday (Mon), Tuesday (Tues), Wednesday
(Wed), Thursday (Thurs), Friday (Fri),
Saturday (Sat), Sunday (Sun)

Telephone phrases

Making a call

Hello/Good morning/Good afternoon.
This is Anna Schwarz from Doctor Hehn's
surgery.
Could I speak to John Baker, please?
Could I please leave him a message?
Could you ask him to call me back, please?

Answering a call

Hello/Good morning/Good afternoon. Dr
Hehn's surgery, Anna Schwarz speaking.
Can I help you?

Could I have your name/address/telephone
number, please?
Could you spell your name, please?
Could I ask who's speaking?
I'm afraid the doctor is busy/not here.
Could I take a message?
Can she call you back?

Making an appointment

I'd like to make an appointment for ... .
Is 2 o'clock on Thursday OK?
What/How about Friday at 10 a.m.?
I'm afraid we close at 4.30 on Mondays.

Finishing a call

OK. See you on ... at ... .
Thanks for calling. Goodbye/Bye.

Saying phone numbers

0 = oh (BE), zero (AE)
190654 = one – nine – oh/zero – six – five – four
276883 = two – seven – six – double eight –
three

The alphabet

	Phonetic code	International code
A	ay	Alpha
B	bee	Bravo
C	see	Charly
D	dee	Delta
E	ee	Echo
F	eff	Foxtrot
G	gee	Golf
H	aytch	Hotel
I	eye	India
J	jay	Juliet
K	kay	Kilo
L	ell	London/Lima

	Phonetic code	International code
M	emm	Mama/Mike
N	enn	November
O	oh	Oscar
P	pee	Papa
Q	queue	Quebec/Queen
R	are	Romeo
S	ess	Sierra
T	tee	Tango
U	you	Uniform
V	vee	Victor
W	double-you	Whisky
X	ex	X-Ray
Y	why	Yankee/Yellow
Z	zed (AE zee)	Zulu

Phonetic:
My name is 'Wills'. That's 'double-you –
eye – double ell – ess'.

International:
My name is 'Wills'. That's 'double-you as in
Whisky – eye as in India – double ell as in
Lima – ess as in Sierra'.

Common irregular verbs

infinitive, simple past, perfect participle

be	was/were – *been*	*sein*
become	became – *become*	*werden*
begin	began – *begun*	*anfangen*
bring	brought – *brought*	*bringen*
build	built – *built*	*bauen*
buy	bought – *bought*	*kaufen*
catch	caught – *caught*	*fangen*
choose	chose – *chosen*	*auswählen*
come	came – *come*	*kommen*
cost	cost – *cost*	*kosten*
cut	cut – *cut*	*schneiden*
do	did – *done*	*tun, machen, erledigen*
draw	drew – *drawn*	*zeichnen*
drink	drank – *drunk*	*trinken, saufen*
drive	drove – *driven*	*fahren*
eat	ate – *eaten*	*essen, fressen*
fall	fell – *fallen*	*hinfallen*
feed	fed – *fed*	*füttern*
feel	felt – *felt*	*sich fühlen*
fight	fought – *fought*	*(be)kämpfen*
find	found – *found*	*finden*
fly	flew – *flown*	*fliegen*
forget	forgot – *forgotten*	*vergessen*
give	gave – *given*	*geben*
get	got – *got*	*bekommen, erhalten*
go	went – *gone*	*gehen*
grow	grew – *grown*	*wachsen*
hang	hung – *hung*	*(auf)hängen*
have	had – *had*	*haben*
hear	heard – *heard*	*hören*
hide	hid – *hidden*	*verstecken*
hit	hit – *hit*	*schlagen, aufprallen auf*
hold	held – *held*	*halten*
hurt	hurt – *hurt*	*verletzen*
keep	kept – *kept*	*behalten*
know	knew – *known*	*kennen, wissen*
lead	led – *led*	*führen, leiten*
leave	left – *left*	*verlassen*
lend	lent – *lent*	*(ver)leihen*
let	let – *let*	*lassen*
light	lit – *lit*	*anzünden*
lose	lost – *lost*	*verlieren*
make	made – *made*	*machen*
mean	meant – *meant*	*bedeuten*
meet	met – *met*	*sich treffen*
pay	paid – *paid*	*(be-)zahlen*
put	put – *put*	*setzen, stellen, legen*

read	read – *read*	*lesen*
ride	rode – *ridden*	*reiten*
ring	rang – *rung*	*klingeln*
rise	rose – *risen*	*steigen*
run	ran – *run*	*laufen*
say	said – *said*	*sagen*
see	saw – *seen*	*sehen*
sell	sold – *sold*	*verkaufen*
send	sent – *sent*	*senden, schicken*
shake	shook – *shaken*	*schütteln*
sing	sang – *sung*	*singen*
sit	sat – *sat*	*sitzen*
speak	spoke – *spoken*	*sprechen*
spend	spent – *spent*	*ausgeben, verbringen*
stand	stood – *stood*	*stehen*
steal	stole – *stolen*	*stehlen*
swim	swam – *swum*	*schwimmen*
take	took – *taken*	*nehmen*
teach	taught – *taught*	*unterrichten, lehren*
tear	tore – *torn*	*(zer)reißen*
tell	told – *told*	*erzählen, mitteilen, sagen*
think	thought – *thought*	*denken, meinen*

throw	threw – *thrown*	*werfen*
understand	understood – *understood*	*verstehen*
wear	wore – *worn*	*tragen, anhaben*
win	won – *won*	*gewinnen*
write	wrote – *written*	*schreiben*

Be careful with:

burn	burnt – burnt	*(ver)brennen*
	burned – burned	
dream	dreamt – dreamt	*träumen*
	dreamed – dreamed	
learn	learnt – learnt	*lernen,*
	learned – learned	*erfahren*
smell	smellt – smellt	*riechen*
	smelled – smelled	
spell	spellt – spellt	*buchstabieren*
	spelled – spelled	
spoil	spoilt – spoilt	*verderben*
	spoiled – spoiled	

Basic word list

Diese Liste enthält 370 Grundwörter, die in Health Matters als bekannt vorausgesetzt werden. Nicht aufgeführt, jedoch vorausgesetzt sind einige elementare Wörter, wie Pronomen, Zahlen, Farben, Wochentage, Monatsnamen sowie Wörter, die im Englischen und Deutschen entweder identisch oder sehr ähnlich sind (z. B. hobby, alcohol, house) oder als Lehnwörter weit verbreitet sind (z. B. job, ticket, phone).

A
a lot viel, sehr
about über, ungefähr
above über, oben, oberhalb
adult Erwachsene/r
after nach, nachdem
afternoon Nachmittag
again wieder
age Alter
all alle
already schon, bereits
also auch, außerdem
always immer
animal Tier
another noch eine/r/s, ein/e andere/r/s
answer Antwort; beantworten

any irgendetwas, irgendwelche/r/s, jede/r/s
anybody jemand, jeder
anyone jemand, jede/r
anywhere irgendwo, irgendwohin
apple Apfel
area Gegend, Umgebung, Gebiet, Bereich
around herum, ungefähr
arrive ankommen
as wie, als
ask fragen, bitten

B
bad schlecht, schlimm
bag Tüte, Tasche
bank Bank, Ufer
basic grundlegend, wesentlich, einfach
be sein
be called heißen
because da, weil
become werden
bed Bett
beer Bier
before vor, vorher
begin anfangen, beginnen
beginning Anfang
between zwischen
big groß, dick

biology Biologie
birthday Geburtstag
black schwarz
book Buch, Heft
both beide
box Kasten
boy Junge
bread Brot
breakfast Frühstück
bring (mit)bringen, holen
Britain Großbritannien
British Brite/Britin; britisch
buy kaufen

C
cake Kuchen
can dürfen, können
car Auto
card Karte
central zentral
chair Stuhl
cheese Käse
child, children Kind, Kinder
chocolate Schokolade, Praline
cigarette Zigarette
cinema Kino
city (Groß-)Stadt
clean sauber; reinigen
climb klettern, steigen
close schließen
coffee Kaffee

cold kalt
colour Farbe
come kommen
contact Kontakt
correct richtig, korrekt; berichtigen, korrigieren
cost Kosten; kosten
could konnte/n, könnte/n
country Land, Staat
cup Tasse
cut schneiden

D
dark, darker dunkel, dunkler
date Datum
daughter Tochter
day Tag
dear liebe/r
department store Warenhaus
do tun, machen
doctor Doktor, Arzt/Ärztin
door Tür
down (nach) unten, herunter
draw zeichnen
drink trinken
drive fahren
dry trocknen

E
each jede/r/s
each other einander, gegenseitig
early, earlier früh, früher
ear Ohr
earring Ohrring
easy einfach, leicht
eat essen
egg Ei
end Ende
energy Energie
evening Abend
ever je(mals), schon (ein)mal
every jede/r/s
everybody jede/r
everything alles
exam Prüfung
excuse me Entschuldigung
exercise book (Schul-)Heft

F
family Familie
far weit (entfernt); weitaus
fast schnell
favourite Lieblings-
feel (sich) fühlen, der Meinung sein
find finden, suchen
fine gut, in Ordnung
finish (be)enden, aufhören (mit)
first erste/r/s, zuerst

food Essen, Nahrung, Lebensmittel
foot, feet Fuß
football Fußball
forget vergessen
form Form; Formular
free kostenlos, frei
friend Freund/in
fruit Obst, Frucht, Früchte
full voll, vollständig
fun Spaß

G
game Spiel
German Deutsche/r; deutsch; Deutsch
Germany Deutschland
get bekommen, werden, gelangen
girl Mädchen
give geben
glass Glas
glasses Brille
go gehen, fahren
good gut
goodbye auf Wiedersehen
grammar Grammatik
great groß; toll, prima
group Gruppe

H
hair Haar/e
half Hälfte, halb
hard schwierig, hart
have haben
hear hören
heavy schwer
help Hilfe; helfen
here hier
Here we go. Los geht's.
high hoch
hold halten, festhalten
holiday Ferien, Urlaub
home Zuhause, Heim
hope Hoffnung; hoffen
hospital Krankenhaus
hot heiß, warm
hour Stunde
how wie
how long wie lange
however jedoch
hungry hungrig
husband Ehemann

I
idea Idee
in front of vor
into in ... hinein
Ireland Irland
Irish Ire/Irin, irisch

K
keep halten, behalten
kitchen Küche
know kennen, wissen

L
language Sprache
large groß
last letzte/r/s
late spät, zu spät
learn lernen, erfahren
leave abfahren, verlassen
left links
leg Bein
less weniger
let erlauben, (zu)lassen
letter Brief, Buchstabe
like mögen, gern haben
line Linie, Zeile
list Liste
listen anhören, zuhören
little klein, wenig
live wohnen, leben
look schauen, (aus)sehen
look for suchen
lots of viel
love Liebe; lieben, sehr gern mögen
lunch Mittagessen

M
magazine Zeitschrift
make machen
male männlich; Mann
many viele
married (to) verheiratet (mit)
maths Mathe(matik) (Schulfach)
may dürfen, können
medium mittlere/r/s, mittel
meet treffen, kennen lernen
metal Metall
milk Milch
mineral water Mineralwasser
money Geld
month Monat
more mehr, weitere/r/s
morning Morgen, Vormittag
most am meisten
mother Mutter
much viel
must müssen

N
near nahe
nearly fast
need brauchen, benötigen
never nie(mals)

new neu
newspaper Zeitung
next nächste/r/s, danach
next to neben
nice nett, schön
night Nacht
not nicht
nothing nichts
now nun, jetzt
number Nummer, Zahl

O

o'clock ... Uhr
office Büro
often oft, häufig
old, older alt, älter
only nur; einzige/r/s
open öffnen; offen
opposite gegenüber
other andere/r/s
over (vor)über

P

paper Papier, Zeitung
parents Eltern
pay (be)zahlen
person, people Mensch(en)
picture Bild
piece Stück
place Ort, Platz
plane Flugzeug
please bitte
point Punkt
popular beliebt
post office Postamt
potato Kartoffel
pound Pfund (Sterling)
present Gegenwart; Geschenk
price (Kauf-)Preis
put setzen, stellen, legen

Q, R

question Frage
quick(ly) schnell
quiet leise, ruhig
read lesen
ready fertig, bereit
really wirklich, eigentlich
right rechts, richtig
road Straße
role Rolle
room Zimmer, Raum

S

salad Salat
salt Salz
same gleiche/r/s, der-, die-,
    dasselbe

say sagen
school Schule
second zweite/r/s
see sehen
sell verkaufen
sentence Satz
shall sollen, werden
shirt Hemd
short, shorter kurz, kürzer
should solle/n, sollte/n
side Seite
sign Zeichen, Anzeichen
silver Silber
sit sitzen
sleep schlafen
slow, slowly langsam
small, smaller klein, kleiner
so also, damit
soft weich
some einige, etwas
somebody jemand
someone jemand
something etwas
sometimes manchmal
somewhere irgendwo, irgend-
    wohin
son Sohn
sorry Entschuldigung; Tut mir
    Leid.
speak sprechen, reden
sport Sport
start anfangen
stay bleiben
stop anhalten, aufhören
story Geschichte
street Straße
strong stark
sugar Zucker
summer Sommer
sweet Bonbon; süß

T

table Tisch; Tabelle
take nehmen, dauern
talk Gespräch; reden
tea Tee
tell sagen, erzählen
thank you danke
thanks Dank; danke
then dann
there da, dort, dorthin
these diese
thing Sache, Ding
think denken, meinen, finden
those jene
through durch, hindurch
time Zeit
today heute

tomorrow morgen
tonight heute Abend/Nacht
top oberer Teil, oberste/r/s
town Stadt
toy Spielzeug
travel reisen

U–V

understand verstehen
unhappy unglücklich
United Kingdom (UK)
    Vereinigtes Königreich
use benutzen, gebrauchen
useful nützlich
vegetables Gemüse
very sehr

W

wait warten
walk Spaziergang; (zu Fuß)
    gehen
wall Wand
want wollen
wash (sich) waschen
water Wasser
wear (Kleidung etc.:) tragen
week Woche
weekday Wochentag
weekend Wochenende
well gut; also
what was, welche/r/s
when wenn, als, wann
where wo, wohin
which welche/r/s
white weiß
who wer, der/die/das
why warum
wife (Ehe-)Frau
will werde(n)
window Fenster
wine Wein
wish wünschen
with mit, bei
without ohne
woman Frau
word Wort
work Arbeit; arbeiten
world Welt
would würde, würdest, würden
write schreiben

Y

year Jahr
yesterday gestern
young, younger jung, jünger

Unit word list

Diese neuen Wörter sind in der Reihenfolge ihres Vorkommens im Text verzeichnet. Es fehlen jedoch die Wörter, die zum Grundwortschatz gehören *(siehe Basic word list)*.
Die Zahl am linken Rand gibt die Seitenzahl an.
T = Das Wort befindet sich im Transkript der Hörverständnistexte.

Unit 1

6	reception [rɪ'sepʃn]	Anmeldung, Rezeption
	surgery ['sɜːdʒəri]	(Arzt-)Praxis
	medical assistant [ˌmedɪkl ə'sɪstənt]	Medizinische Fach-angestellte/r
	appointment [ə'pɔɪntmənt]	Termin
	Don't worry. [dəʊnt 'wʌri]	Keine Sorge.
	be busy [bi 'bɪzi]	viel zu tun haben
	fit sb in [ˌfɪt 'ɪn]	jdn dazwischenschieben
	health [helθ]	Gesundheit
	health insurance ['helθ ɪnʃʊərəns]	Krankenversicherung
	insurance card [ɪn'ʃʊərəns kɑːd]	Versichertenkarte
	surgery charge ['sɜːdʒəri tʃɑːdʒ]	Praxisgebühr
	receipt [rɪ'siːt]	Quittung, Beleg
	You're welcome. [jɔː 'welkəm]	Bitte. Gern geschehen.
	take a seat [ˌteɪk ə 'siːt]	Platz nehmen
	waiting room ['weɪtɪŋ ruːm]	Wartezimmer
	statement ['steɪtmənt]	Aussage, Behauptung
	true [truː]	wahr
	false [fɔːls]	falsch
	immediately [ɪ'miːdiətli]	sofort
	culture ['kʌltʃə]	Kultur
	politeness [pə'laɪtnəs]	Höflichkeit
	inconvenience sb [ˌɪnkən'viːniəns]	jdm Umstände bereiten
	response [rɪ'spɒns]	Antwort
7	manage ['mænɪdʒ]	schaffen, einrichten
	a quarter to [ə 'kwɔːtə tə]	Viertel vor
	a quarter past [ə 'kwɔːtə pɑːst]	Viertel nach
	match [mætʃ]	zuordnen
	phone call ['fəʊn kɔːl]	Telefongespräch, Anruf
	caller ['kɔːlə]	Anrufer/in
	health centre ['helθ sentə]	Gesundheitszentrum T
	certainly ['sɜːtnli]	sicherlich T
	particular [pə'tɪkjələ]	spezielle/r/s T

	prefer [prɪ'fɜː]	vorziehen, (lieber) mögen T
	appointment book [ə'pɔɪntmənt bʊk]	Terminkalender T
8	patient ['peɪʃnt]	Patient/in
	I'm fine. [aɪm 'faɪn]	Mir geht es gut.
	pain [peɪn]	Schmerz, Schmerzen
	be in pain [ˌbi ɪn 'peɪn]	Schmerzen haben
	prescription [prɪ'skrɪpʃn]	Rezept
	practice ['præktɪs]	Übung, Training
	result [rɪ'zʌlt]	Ergebnis, Resultat
	blood [blʌd]	Blut
	blood test ['blʌd test]	Blutuntersuchung
	spell [spel]	buchstabieren
	choose [tʃuːz]	wählen
	spelling ['spelɪŋ]	Schreibweise
9	deal with sb ['diːl wɪð]	mit jdm umgehen, sich um jdn kümmern
	Australian [ɒ'streɪliən]	Australier/in
	below [bɪ'ləʊ]	unten(stehend)
	health care ['helθ keə]	Gesundheitswesen
	General Practitioner [ˌdʒenrəl præk'tɪʃənə]	Allgemeinarzt/-ärztin
	register (with sb) ['redʒɪstə]	sich (bei jdm) anmelden
	in order to [ɪn'ɔːdə tə]	um ... zu
	receive [rɪ'siːv]	erhalten, bekommen
	health care ['helθ keə]	medizinische Versor-gung
	move house [ˌmuːv 'haʊs]	umziehen
	practise ['præktɪs]	üben
	similar ['sɪmələ]	ähnlich
	postcode ['pəʊstkəʊd]	Postleitzahl
	need to do sth [ˌniːd tə 'duː]	etw tun müssen
	practice ['præktɪs]	Praxis
	complete [kəm'pliːt]	ausfüllen
	medical history [ˌmedɪkl 'hɪstri]	Krankengeschichte
	form [fɔːm]	Formular
	have a look [həv ə 'lʊk]	nachschauen
	details ['diːteɪlz]	Angaben, Einzelheiten
10	patient record file [ˌpeɪʃnt 'rekɔːd faɪl]	Patientenakte, Kranken-akte
	copy ['kɒpi]	abschreiben
	missing ['mɪsɪŋ]	fehlend
	personal details [ˌpɜːsnəl 'diːteɪlz]	persönliche Angaben
	complete [kəm'pliːt]	vervollständigen
	role play ['rəʊl pleɪ]	mit verteilten Rollen spielen

11 material [mə'tɪərɪəl]   Material
    medical receptionist   Sprechstundenhilfe
       [ˌmedɪkl rɪ'sepʃənɪst]
    training ['treɪnɪŋ]   Ausbildung
    leaflet ['liːflət]   Broschüre, Merkblatt
    note [nəʊt]   notieren, aufschreiben
    important [ɪm'pɔːtnt]   wichtig, bedeutend
    qualification   Abschluss, Qualifikation,
       [ˌkwɒlɪfɪ'keɪʃn]   Voraussetzung
    summarize ['sʌməraɪz]   zusammenfassen
    difference ['dɪfrəns]   Unterschied
    intermediate diploma   Zwischenprüfung
       [ˌɪntəˌmiːdiət dɪ'pləʊmə]
    caring ['keərɪŋ]   sozial (eingestellt)
    enjoy doing sth [ɪn'dʒɔɪ]   etw gern tun
    part [pɑːt]   Teil
    medical administration   medizinische Verwal-
       [ˌmedɪkl ədmɪnɪ'streɪʃn]   tungsaufgaben
    within [wɪ'ðɪn]   innerhalb
    environment   Umfeld, Umgebung
       [ɪn'vaɪrənmənt]
    front line [ˌfrʌnt 'laɪn]   *etwa:* an vorderster
          Front
    staff [stɑːf]   Personal
    relative ['relətɪv]   Verwandte/r
    either ... or ['aɪðə ɔː]   entweder ... oder
    in person [ɪn 'pɜːsn]   persönlich
    involved in [ɪn'vɒlvd ɪn]   beteiligt an
    book [bʊk]   buchen
    scheme [skiːm]   Programm, Projekt, Plan
    impression [ɪm'preʃn]   Eindruck
    affect [ə'fekt]   beeinflussen
    opinion [ə'pɪnɪən]   Meinung, Ansicht
    general practice   Allgemeinarztpraxis
       [ˌdʒenrəl 'præktɪs]
    study for sth ['stʌdi fə]   für etw lernen
    knowledge ['nɒlɪdʒ]   Wissen, Kenntnisse
    skills [skɪlz]   Fertigkeiten, Fähigkeiten
    required [rɪ'kwaɪəd]   erforderlich, nötig
    interesting ['ɪntrəstɪŋ]   interessant
    challenging ['tʃælɪndʒɪŋ]   fordernd, anspruchsvoll
    achieve [ə'tʃiːv]   erreichen, erlangen
    diploma [dɪ'pləʊmə]   Diplom
    gain a pass [ˌgeɪn ə 'pɑːs]   eine Prüfung bestehen
    written ['rɪtn]   schriftlich
    examination/exam   Prüfung
       [ɪgˌzæmɪ'neɪʃn/ɪg'zæm]
    assignment [ə'saɪnmənt]   Aufgabe
    nationally set   landesweit einheitlich
       [ˌnæʃnəli 'set]
    satisfy requirements   Bedingungen erfüllen
       [ˌsætɪsfaɪ rɪ'kwaɪəmənts]
    work experience   Berufs-/Arbeitserfah-
       ['wɜːk ɪkspɪərɪəns]   rung
    pass [pɑːs]   *(Prüfung)* bestehen
    work-based assignment   praktische Prüfungs-
       [ˌwɜːk beɪst ə'saɪnmənt]   aufgabe
    available [ə'veɪləbl]   verfügbar, erhältlich

    full time [ˌfʊl 'taɪm]   Vollzeit-
    part time [ˌpɑːt 'taɪm]   Teilzeit-
    study ['stʌdi]   Studium, Ausbildung
    average ['ævərɪdʒ]   Durchschnitt, Durch-
          schnitts-
    length [leŋθ]   Länge
    course [kɔːs]   Kurs
    suitable ['suːtəbl]   geeignet
    both ... and [bəʊθ ənd]   sowohl ... als auch
    school leaver [ˌskuːl liːvə]   Schulabgänger/in
    mature [mə'tʃʊə]   hier: ältere
    member ['membə]   Mitglied
    feeling ['fiːlɪŋ]   Gefühl

Unit 2

12 typical ['tɪpɪkl]   typisch
    activity [æk'tɪvəti]   Tätigkeit
    nurse [nɜːs]   Krankenschwester/
          -pfleger
    radiologist   Radiologe/-in
       [ˌreɪdi'ɒlədʒɪst]
    paediatrician   Kinderarzt/-ärztin
       [ˌpiːdiə'trɪʃn]
    physiotherapist   Physiotherapeut/in
       [ˌfɪziəʊ'θerəpɪst]
    gynaecologist   Gynäkologe/-in
       [ˌgaɪnə'kɒlədʒɪst]
    X-rays ['eksreɪz]   Röntgenstrahlen
    take X-rays [ˌteɪk 'eksreɪz]   röntgen
    check-up ['tʃekʌp]   (Vorsorge-)Untersu-
          chung
    assist sb [ə'sɪst]   jdm assistieren
    joint [dʒɔɪnt]   Gelenk
    movement ['muːvmənt]   Bewegung
    specialize ['speʃəlaɪz]   sich spezialisieren
    treat [triːt]   behandeln
    diagnose ['daɪəgnəʊz]   diagnostizieren
    general ['dʒenrəl]   allgemein
    treatment room   Behandlungszimmer
       ['triːtmənt rʊm]
    sterilization   Sterilisation
       [ˌsterəlaɪ'zeɪʃn]
    staffroom ['stɑːfrʊm]   Personalraum
    laboratory/lab   Labor
       [lə'bɒrətri/læb]

13 description [dɪ'skrɪpʃn]   Beschreibung
    community [kə'mjuːnəti]   Gemeinde
    job opening   offene Stelle, Stellen-
       ['dʒɒb əʊpnɪŋ]   angebot
    following ['fɒləʊɪŋ]   folgende/r/s
    outgoing ['aʊtgəʊɪŋ]   kontaktfreudig
    personality [ˌpɜːsə'næləti]   Persönlichkeit
    ability [ə'bɪləti]   Fähigkeit
    supportive [sə'pɔːtɪv]   hilfreich, verständnisvoll
    manner ['mænə]   Art (und Weise)
    background ['bækgraʊnd]   Herkunft, Hintergrund
    excellent ['eksələnt]   ausgezeichnet

pressure ['preʃə]	Druck	14	complete [kəm'pli:t]	vollständig
accurate ['ækjərət]	genau, akkurat		records ['rekɔ:dz]	Aufzeichnungen,
efficient [ɪ'fɪʃnt]	effizient			Unterlagen
experience [ɪk'spɪərɪəns]	Erfahrung		keep records	Aufzeichnungen führen,
duties ['dju:tiz]	Aufgaben		[ˌki:p 'rekɔ:dz]	Akten halten
include [ɪn'klu:d]	einschließen, beinhalten		visit ['vɪzɪt]	besuchen
greet [gri:t]	begrüßen		supplies [sə'plaɪz]	Artikel, Bedarf, Vorräte
polite [pə'laɪt]	höflich		medical supplies	Sanitätsartikel
helpful ['helpfl]	hilfsbereit		[ˌmedɪkl sə'plaɪz]	
public ['pʌblɪk]	Publikum		usually ['ju:ʒuəli]	normalerweise, gewöhn-
respect [rɪ'spekt]	respektieren			lich
privacy ['prɪvəsi]	Privatsphäre		injection [ɪn'dʒekʃn]	Injektion, Spritze
dignity ['dɪgnəti]	Würde		describe [dɪ'skraɪb]	beschreiben
provide [prə'vaɪd]	bieten		medical practice	Arztpraxis
service ['sɜ:vɪs]	Dienst, Dienstleistung		[ˌmedɪkl 'præktɪs]	
register sb ['redʒɪstə]	jdn registrieren,			
	aufnehmen	15	equipment [ɪ'kwɪpmənt]	Ausstattung, Geräte
fee [fi:]	Honorar, Gebühr		illustration [ˌɪlə'streɪʃn]	Abbildung
collect [kə'lekt]	sammeln, kassieren		appointment card	Terminzettel
payment ['peɪmənt]	Zahlung		[ə'pɔɪntmənt kɑ:d]	
order ['ɔ:də]	bestellen		calendar ['kælɪndə]	Kalender
office supplies	Bürobedarf		card reader port	Kartenlesegerät
['ɒfɪs səplaɪz]			['kɑ:d ri:də pɔ:t]	
front desk [ˌfrʌnt 'desk]	Rezeption, Anmeldung		cash box ['kæʃ bɒks]	Kasse
close [kləʊz]	schließen, abschließen		printer ['prɪntə]	Drucker
building ['bɪldɪŋ]	Gebäude		date stamp ['deɪt stæmp]	Datumsstempel
working day ['wɜ:kɪŋ deɪ]	Arbeitstag		fax machine	Fax(gerät)
turn off [ˌtɜ:n 'ɒf]	ab-/ausschalten		['fæks məʃi:n]	
unplug sth [ˌʌn'plʌg]	den Stecker von etw		filing cabinet	Aktenschrank
	herausziehen		['faɪlɪŋ kæbɪnət]	
appliance [ə'plaɪəns]	Gerät		inkpad ['ɪŋkpæd]	Stempelkissen
machine [mə'ʃi:n]	Gerät, Maschine		label printer	Etikettendrucker
ready for business	betriebsbereit		['leɪbl prɪntə]	
[ˌredi fə 'bɪznəs]			memo pad ['meməʊ pæd]	Notizzettelblock
take part in sth	an etw teilnehmen		paper clip ['peɪpə klɪp]	Büroklammer
[ˌteɪk 'pɑ:t ɪn]			scissors ['sɪzəz]	Schere
educational	Ausbildungs-		stapler ['steɪplə]	Heftgerät, Tacker
[ˌedʒu'keɪʃnəl]			suspended pocket file	Hängesammler, Hänge-
meeting ['mi:tɪŋ]	Sitzung, Besprechung,		[sə,spendɪd 'pɒkɪt faɪl]	register
	Treffen		store [stɔ:]	lagern
rank [ræŋk]	einstufen		note [nəʊt]	Notiz
order ['ɔ:də]	Reihenfolge		ink [ɪŋk]	einfärben
importance [ɪm'pɔ:tns]	Bedeutung, Wichtigkeit		file [faɪl]	(Akten) ablegen
add [æd]	hinzufügen		fix [fɪks]	befestigen
personnel [ˌpɜ:sə'nel]	Personal		print [prɪnt]	ausdrucken
administrative staff	Verwaltungspersonal		label ['leɪbl]	Etikett
[əd,mɪnɪstrətɪv 'stɑ:f]			stamp [stæmp]	stempeln
train [treɪn]	ausbilden		send [send]	(ver)senden, (ver)-
legally ['li:gəli]	gesetzlich, von Gesetzes			schicken
	wegen		attach [ə'tætʃ]	befestigen
be allowed to do sth	etw tun dürfen			
[bi ə'laʊd tə]		16	give directions	den Weg beschreiben
clinical ['klɪnɪkl]	klinisch		[gɪv də'rekʃnz]	
qualified ['kwɒlɪfaɪd]	ausgebildet, qualifiziert		storeroom ['stɔ:ru:m]	Lagerraum
state [steɪt]	Staat, Land		key [ki:]	Schlüssel T
present ['preznt]	anwesend, zugegen		turn left/right	links/rechts abbiegen T
			[ˌtɜ:n 'left/'raɪt]	
			corridor ['kɒrɪdɔ:]	Flur T

show [ʃəʊ]	zeigen T	
ID (card) [ˌaɪ 'diː ˈkɑːd]	Personalausweis T	
delivery [dɪˈlɪvəri]	Lieferung T	
delivery note [dɪˈlɪvəri nəʊt]	Lieferschein T	
check [tʃek]	überprüfen T	
sign [saɪn]	unterschreiben T	
pharmaceutical [ˌfɑːməˈsuːtɪkl]	pharmazeutisch, Pharma- T	
company [ˈkʌmpəni]	Gesellschaft, Firma T	
label [ˈleɪbl]	beschriften T	
straight on [ˌstreɪt ˈɒn]	geradeaus	
stairs [steəz]	Treppe	

17 foreign [ˈfɒrən] — ausländisch
visitor [ˈvɪzɪtə] — Besucher/in
translate [trænsˈleɪt] — übersetzen
questionnaire [ˌkwestʃəˈneə] — Fragebogen
dictionary [ˈdɪkʃənri] — Wörterbuch
medical [ˈmedɪkl] — medizinisch, ärztlich
allergic [əˈlɜːdʒɪk] — allergisch
reaction [riˈækʃn] — Reaktion
drug [drʌg] — Arzneimittel, Medikament
tablet [ˈtæblɪt] — Tablette
medicine [ˈmedsn] — Arzneimittel
pregnant [ˈpregnənt] — schwanger
hepatitis [ˌhepəˈtaɪtɪs] — Hepatitis
anxious [ˈæŋkʃəs] — besorgt, ängstlich, nervös
kind [kaɪnd] — Art T
anaesthetic [ˌænəsˈθetɪk] — Betäubungsmittel T
medication [ˌmedɪˈkeɪʃn] — Medikamente T
finally [ˈfaɪnəli] — zuletzt, als letztes T
nervous [ˈnɜːvəs] — nervös T

Unit 3

18 symptom [ˈsɪmptəm] — Symptom
different [ˈdɪfrənt] — verschieden, unterschiedlich
break [breɪk] — brechen; Bruch
crutches [ˈkrʌtʃɪz] — Krücken
almost [ˈɔːlməʊst] — fast, beinah
sure [ʃʊə] — sicher
deaf [def] — taub
ear wax [ˈɪə wæks] — Ohrenschmalz
syringe [sɪˈrɪndʒ] — *(Ohr etc.)* ausspülen
migraine [ˈmiːgreɪn] — Migräne
head [hed] — Kopf
cut your arm [ˌkʌt jɔːr ˈɑːm] — sich in den Arm schneiden
repair [rɪˈpeə] — reparieren
bike [baɪk] — Fahrrad
cut [kʌt] — Schnitt, Schnittverletzung
near [nɪə] — nahe
close by [ˌkləʊs ˈbaɪ] — nahe gelegen

straight away [streɪt əˈweɪ] — sofort
smear test [ˈsmɪə test] — Abstrich
routine test [ruːˈtiːn test] — Routineuntersuchung
regular [ˈregjələ] — regelmäßig
illness [ˈɪlnəs] — Krankheit
exercise [ˈeksəsaɪz] — trainieren
muscle [ˈmʌsl] — Muskel
specialist [ˈspeʃəlɪst] — Facharzt/-ärztin

19 chest [tʃest] — Brust
infection [ɪnˈfekʃn] — Infektion
antibiotics [ˌæntibaɪˈɒtɪks] — Antibiotika

20 be careful of sth [bi ˈkeəfl əv] — auf etw achten, auf etw. aufpassen
negative [ˈnegətɪv] — Verneinung
visit [ˈvɪzɪt] — Besuch
move [muːv] — umziehen
village [ˈvɪlɪdʒ] — Dorf
mile [maɪl] — Meile
called [kɔːld] — namens
tray [treɪ] — Schale
hurt [hɜːt] — wehtun
at all [ət ˈɔːl] — überhaupt
still [stɪl] — (immer) noch
apply for sth [əˈplaɪ fə] — sich um etw bewerben
leave school [ˌliːv ˈskuːl] — von der Schule abgehen
comfortable [ˈkʌmftəbl] — angenehm
painful [ˈpeɪnfl] — schmerzhaft
acronym [ˈækrənɪm] — Abkürzung, Akronym
nose [nəʊz] — Nase
throat [θrəʊt] — Rachen, Hals
electrocardiograph [ɪˌlektrəʊˈkɑːdiəʊgrɑːf] — Elektrokardiogramm
measure [ˈmeʒə] — messen
electrical [ɪˈlektrɪkl] — elektrisch
charge [tʃɑːdʒ] — Ladung
heart [hɑːt] — Herz
electroencephalograph [ɪˌlektrəʊɪnˈsefələgrɑːf] — Elektroenzephalogramm
brain [breɪn] — Gehirn, Hirn
electromyogram [ɪˌlektrəʊˈmaɪəgræm] — Elektromyogramm

21 highlight [ˈhaɪlaɪt] — hervorheben
diagram [ˈdaɪəgræm] — Grafik
outer ear [ˌaʊtər ˈɪə] — Außenohr
cartilage [ˈkɑːtɪlɪdʒ] — Knorpel
outside [ˌaʊtˈsaɪd] — Außenseite
channel sth [ˈtʃænl] — etw leiten
sound wave [ˈsaʊnd weɪv] — Schallwelle
external [ɪkˈstɜːnl] — äußere/r/s
ear canal [ˌɪə kəˈnæl] — Gehörgang
eardrum [ˈɪədrʌm] — Trommelfell
separate [ˈseprət] — trennen
middle ear [ˌmɪdl ˈɪə] — Mittelohr

turn sth into sth [ˈtɜːn ˌɪntə]	etw in etw umwandeln
amplify [ˈæmplɪfaɪ]	verstärken
ossicles [ˈɒsɪklz]	Gehörknöchelchen
chain [tʃeɪn]	Kette
tiny [ˈtaɪni]	winzig
bone [bəʊn]	Knochen
anvil [ˈænvɪl]	Amboss
stirrup [ˈstɪrəp]	Steigbügel
inner ear [ˌɪnər ˈɪə]	Innenohr
cochlea [ˈkɒkliə]	Hörschnecke
auditory nerve [ˌɒdətri ˈnɜːv]	Hörnerv
semi-circular canals [semiˌsɜːkjələ kəˈnælz]	Bogengänge
fluid [ˈfluːɪd]	Flüssigkeit
filled [fɪld]	gefüllt
control [kənˈtrəʊl]	kontrollieren
balance [ˈbæləns]	Gleichgewicht
Eustachian tube [juːˌsteɪʃn ˈtjuːb]	Eustachi-Röhre
connect [kəˈnekt]	verbinden
pop [pɒp]	ploppen
mouth [maʊθ]	Mund
trainee [treɪˈniː]	Auszubildende/r
heading [ˈhedɪŋ]	Überschrift
nasal passage [ˌneɪzl ˈpæsɪdʒ]	Nasengang
olfactory nerve [ɒlˌfæktəri ˈnɜːv]	Geruchsnerv
windpipe [ˈwɪndpaɪp]	Luftröhre
trachea [trəˈkiə]	Trachea
palate [ˈpælət]	Gaumen
tongue [tʌŋ]	Zunge
gullet [ˈgʌlɪt]	Speiseröhre
oesophagus [iˈsɒfəgəs]	Oesophagus
name [neɪm]	nennen, benennen
explain [ɪkˈspleɪn]	erklären, erläutern
function [ˈfʌŋkʃn]	Funktion
finished [ˈfɪnɪʃt]	fertig T
together (with) [təˈgeðə wɪð]	zusammen (mit) T
of course [əf ˈkɔːs]	natürlich T
passage [ˈpæsɪdʒ]	Gang, Weg T
air [eə]	Luft T
body [ˈbɒdi]	Körper T
take in (air) [teɪk ˌɪn ˈeə]	(Luft) einatmen T
pass over sth [ˌpɑːs ˈəʊvə]	*hier:* über etw streichen T
back [bæk]	Rückseite, hinterer Teil T
carry [ˈkæri]	befördern T
lungs [lʌŋz]	Lunge T
tooth, teeth [tuːθ, tiːθ]	Zahn, Zähne T
lip [lɪp]	Lippe T
front [frʌnt]	Vorderseite, vorderer Teil T
middle [ˈmɪdl]	Mitte, mittlerer Teil T

roof [ruːf]	Dach T
major [ˈmeɪdʒə]	Haupt- T
organ [ˈɔːgən]	Organ T
taste [teɪst]	Geschmack T
remember [rɪˈmembə]	denken an, nicht vergessen T
smell [smel]	Geruch T
way [weɪ]	Art (und Weise) T
taste [teɪst]	schmecken T
anyway [ˈeniweɪ]	also, wie dem auch sei T
swallow [ˈswɒləʊ]	schlucken T
tube [tjuːb]	Röhre T
stomach [ˈstʌmək]	Magen T

22
make a diagnosis [ˌmeɪk ə daɪəgˈnəʊsɪs]	eine Diagnose stellen
sore throat [ˌsɔː ˈθrəʊt]	Halsschmerzen
sore [sɔː]	wund
wide [waɪd]	weit
trouble [ˈtrʌbl]	Schwierigkeit(en), Problem(e)
thermometer [θəˈmɒmɪtə]	Thermometer
take one's temperature [teɪk ˈtemprətʃə]	bei jdm Fieber messen
high [haɪ]	*hier:* erhöht
gland [glænd]	Drüse
swollen [ˈswəʊlən]	geschwollen
breathe [briːð]	atmen
tired [ˈtaɪəd]	müde
tonsils [ˈtɒnslz]	Mandeln
inflamed [ɪnˈfleɪmd]	entzündet
probably [ˈprɒbəbli]	wahrscheinlich
tonsillitis [ˌtɒnsəˈlaɪtɪs]	Mandelentzündung
swab [swɒb]	Tupfer; Abstrich
find out [ˌfaɪnd ˈaʊt]	herausfinden
cause [kɔːz]	verursachen
prescribe [prɪˈskraɪb]	verschreiben, verordnen
plenty of [ˈplenti əv]	viel(e)
rest [rest]	Ruhe
get some rest [ˌget səm ˈrest]	sich ausruhen
sick note [ˈsɪk nəʊt]	Krankschreibung, Attest
seem [siːm]	scheinen
neck [nek]	Hals, Nacken
ache [eɪk]	schmerzen

23
temperature [ˈtemprətʃə]	Fieber T
terrible [ˈterəbl]	fürchterlich T
sneeze [sniːz]	niesen T
blocked [blɒkt]	verstopft T
cough [kɒf]	husten T
shoulder [ˈʃəʊldə]	Schulter T
sit down [ˌsɪt ˈdaʊn]	sich (hin)setzen T
vomit [ˈvɒmɪt]	sich erbrechen T
fever [ˈfiːvə]	Fieber T
diarrhoea [ˌdaɪəˈrɪə]	Durchfall T
notice [ˈnəʊtɪs]	bemerken T

pretty ['prɪti]	hübsch T	**keep food down**	Nahrung bei sich be-
shy [ʃaɪ]	schüchtern T	[kiːp ˌfuːd 'daʊn]	halten
Never mind.	Macht nichts. T	**guess** [gɛs]	raten, erraten
[ˌnevə 'maɪnd]			
headache ['hedeɪk]	Kopfschmerzen T	25 **article** ['ɑːtɪkl]	Artikel
rash [ræʃ]	Ausschlag T	**heart disease** ['hɑːt dɪziːz]	Herzerkrankung
spot [spɒt]	Punkt, Fleck T	**die** [daɪ]	sterben
cough [kɒf]	Husten T	**recognise** ['rekəgnaɪz]	erkennen
discuss [dɪ'skʌs]	diskutieren, erörtern	**warning sign**	Warnsignal
poisoning ['pɔɪzənɪŋ]	Vergiftung	['wɔːnɪŋ saɪn]	
food poisoning	Lebensmittelvergiftung	**discover** [dɪ'skʌvə]	entdecken, herausfinden
['fuːd pɔɪzənɪŋ]		**tend** [tend]	dazu neigen
flu / influenza	Grippe	**stressed-out** [ˌstrest 'aʊt]	gestresst
[fluː /ˌɪnflu'enzə]		**overweight** [ˌəʊvə'weɪt]	übergewichtig
measles ['miːzlz]	Masern	**wake-up call**	Weckruf
agree [ə'griː]	zustimmen	['weɪkʌp kɔːl]	
disagree [ˌdɪsə'griː]	nicht zustimmen	**across Europe**	in ganz Europa
local ['ləʊkl]	ortsansässig	[əkrɒs 'jʊərəp]	
National Health Service	Nationaler Gesundheits-	**per cent** [pə 'sent]	Prozent
[ˌnæʃnəl 'helθ sɜːvɪs]	dienst	**compared with**	verglichen mit
cardiologist	Kardiologe/-in	[kəm'peəd wɪð]	
[ˌkɑːdi'ɒlədʒɪst]		**suffer from sth**	an etw leiden
study ['stʌdi]	studieren; untersuchen	['sʌfə frəm]	
disease [dɪ'ziːz]	Krankheit	**mild** [maɪld]	leicht
consultant [kən'sʌltənt]	Facharzt/-ärztin	**heart attack** ['hɑːt ətæk]	Herzinfarkt
senior ['siːniə]	älter, ranghöher	**flight of stairs**	Treppe
complete [kəm'pliːt]	abschließen	[ˌflaɪt əv 'steəz]	
specialist register	Facharztregister	**breath** [breθ]	Atem
['speʃəlɪst redʒɪstə]		**catch one's breath**	Luft/Atem holen
		[ˌkætʃ wʌnz 'breθ]	
24 **examine** [ɪg'zæmɪn]	untersuchen	**dizzy** ['dɪzi]	schwindlig
take (it in) turns	sich abwechseln	**weak** [wiːk]	schwach
[ˌteɪk ɪt ɪn 'tɜːnz]		**severe** [sɪ'vɪə]	*(Schmerzen:)* heftig
sleeve [sliːv]	Ärmel T	**pulse** [pʌls]	Puls
roll up [ˌrəʊl 'ʌp]	*(Ärmel)* hochkrem-	**take sb's pulse**	jds Puls messen
	peln T	[ˌteɪk 'pʌls]	
happen ['hæpən]	passieren, geschehen T	**heart rate** ['hɑːt reɪt]	Puls, Herzfrequenz
try [traɪ]	versuchen T	**skip** [skɪp]	Aussetzer, Unregel-
screwdriver ['skruːdraɪvə]	Schraubenzieher T		mäßigkeit
slip [slɪp]	abrutschen T	**carry out** [ˌkæri 'aʊt]	durchführen
bandage ['bændɪdʒ]	Verband T	**ambulance** ['æmbjələns]	Rettungswagen
long [lɒŋ]	lang T	**call** [kɔːl]	rufen
deep [diːp]	tief T	**calm** [kɑːm]	ruhig
heal [hiːl]	heilen, verheilen T	**stay** [steɪ]	bleiben
stitch [stɪtʃ]	Stich T	**extreme** [ɪk'striːm]	Extrem
recently ['riːsntli]	in letzter Zeit T	**awareness** [ə'weənəs]	Bewusstsein
remember [rɪ'membə]	sich erinnern T	**increase** [ɪn'kriːs]	zunehmen
exactly [ɪg'zæktli]	genau T	**amongst** [ə'mʌŋst]	unter, bei
disinfect [ˌdɪsɪn'fekt]	desinfizieren T	**conscious** ['kɒnʃəs]	bewusst
hold out [ˌhəʊld 'aʊt]	hinhalten T	**considerable**	erheblich
stitch [stɪtʃ]	nähen	[kən'sɪdərəbl]	
consult [kən'sʌlt]	konsultieren; beraten	**lack** [læk]	Mangel
dressing ['dresɪŋ]	Verband	**on the part of**	auf Seiten der
blister ['blɪstə]	Blase	[ɒn ðə 'pɑːt əv]	
scratch [skrætʃ]	Kratzer, Kratzwunde	**director** [də'rektə]	Direktor/in
bruise [bruːz]	blauer Fleck, Prellung	**foundation** [faʊn'deɪʃn]	Stiftung
earache ['ɪəreɪk]	Ohrenschmerzen	**view** [vjuː]	Ansicht
backache ['bækeɪk]	Rückenschmerzen	**reason** ['riːzn]	Grund

mainly ['meɪnli]	hauptsächlich	**take out stitches**	Fäden ziehen
coronary heart disease	koronare Herzerkran-	[teɪk ˌaʊt 'stɪtʃɪz]	
[ˌkɒrənrɪ 'hɑːt dɪziːz]	kung	**tie off stitches**	Fäden verknoten
believe [bɪ'liːv]	glauben	[taɪ ˌɒf 'stɪtʃɪz]	
stressed [strest]	gestresst	**finally** ['faɪnəli]	schließlich, zum Schluss
overworked [ˌəʊvə'wɜːkt]	überarbeitet	**return** [rɪ'tɜːn]	zurückkehren, wieder-
deal with ['diːl wɪð]	zu tun haben mit		kommen
life, lives [laɪf, laɪvz]	Leben	**a couple of** [ə 'kʌpl əv]	ein paar
quite [kwaɪt]	ziemlich	**take effect** [ˌteɪk ɪ'fekt]	wirken, Wirkung zeigen
smoke [sməʊk]	rauchen	**procedure** [prə'siːdʒə]	Vorgang, Verfahren
likely ['laɪkli]	wahrscheinlich		(sweise)
contribute [kən'trɪbjuːt]	beitragen	**reassure sb** [ˌriːə'ʃʊə]	jdn beruhigen
design [dɪ'zaɪn]	gestalten, entwerfen	**sting** [stɪŋ]	schmerzen, brennen T
		hardly ['hɑːdli]	kaum T
Unit 4		**direction** [də'rekʃn]	Richtung T
		light [laɪt]	leicht
26 **identify** [aɪ'dentɪfaɪ]	identifizieren, erkennen,	**relax** [rɪ'læks]	sich entspannen
	benennen	**sympathetic**	mitfühlend, verständnis-
gloves [glʌvz]	Handschuhe	[ˌsɪmpə'θetɪk]	voll
hypodermic (syringe)	(Injektions-)Spritze	**response** [rɪ'spɒns]	Antwort, Reaktion
[haɪpə͵dɜːmɪk sɪ'rɪndʒ]		**wonderful** ['wʌndəfl]	wunderbar
disinfectant	Desinfektionsmittel		
[ˌdɪsɪn'fektənt]		28 **take blood** [ˌteɪk 'blʌd]	Blut abnehmen
elastic bandage	elastische Binde	**immunization**	Impfung, Immunisie-
[ɪˌlæstɪk 'bændɪdʒ]		[ˌɪmjunaɪ'zeɪʃn]	rung
tourniquet ['tʊənɪkeɪ]	Venenstauer	**blood sample**	Blutprobe
tweezers ['twiːzəz]	Pinzette	['blʌd sɑːmpl]	
gauze dressing	Mull-, Gazeverband	**take off** [ˌteɪk 'ɒf]	*(Kleidung)* ausziehen
[ˌgɔːz 'dresɪŋ]		**jacket** ['dʒækɪt]	Jacke
cotton ['kɒtn]	Baumwolle	**tight** [taɪt]	eng, fest
cotton swab [ˌkɒtn 'swɒb]	Wattetupfer	**plaster** ['plɑːstə]	Pflaster
scalpel ['skælpəl]	Skalpell	**actual** ['æktʃuəl]	wirklich, tatsächlich
stethoscope ['steθəskəʊp]	Stethoskop	**sight** [saɪt]	Anblick T
otoscope ['əʊtəʊskəʊp]	Otoskop	**glad** [glæd]	froh T
blood pressure	Blutdruck	**cottonwool** [ˌkɒtn'wʊl]	Watte T
['blʌd preʃə]			
blood-pressure cuff	Blutdruckmanschette	29 **take blood pressure**	den Blutdruck messen
[ˌblʌd preʃə 'kʌf]		[ˌteɪk 'blʌd preʃə]	
surgical needle-holder	Operationsnadelhalter		
[ˌsɜːdʒɪkl 'niːdl həʊldə]		30 **part of the body**	Körperteil
needle-thread combi-	Nadel-Faden-Kombi-	[ˌpɑːt əv ðə 'bɒdi]	
nation	nation	**ankle** ['æŋkl]	(Fuß-)Knöchel
[ˌniːdl 'θred kɒmbɪneɪʃn]		**appendix** [ə'pendɪks]	Blinddarm
piece of equipment	Ausrüstungsgegenstand	**back** [bæk]	Rücken
[ˌpiːs əv ɪ'kwɪpmənt]		**buttocks** ['bʌtəks]	Gesäß, Hinterbacken
dress a wound	eine Wunde verbinden	**chin** [tʃɪn]	Kinn
[ˌdres ə 'wuːnd]		**shin** [ʃɪn]	Schienbein
extract [ɪk'strækt]	herausziehen	**elbow** ['elbəʊ]	Ellbogen
inject [ɪn'dʒekt]	injizieren	**hip** [hɪp]	Hüfte
protect [prə'tekt]	schützen	**jaw** [dʒɔː]	Kiefer
heartbeat ['hɑːtbiːt]	Herzschlag	**kidney** ['kɪdni]	Niere
sprain [spreɪn]	Verstauchung	**knee** [niː]	Knie
splinter ['splɪntə]	Splitter	**liver** ['lɪvə]	Leber
skin [skɪn]	Haut	**thigh** [θaɪ]	Oberschenkel
broken ['brəʊkən]	ge-, zerbrochen	**wrist** [rɪst]	Handgelenk
		knuckle ['nʌkl]	(Finger-)Knöchel
27 **step** [step]	Schritt	**spleen** [spliːn]	Milz
local anaesthetic	örtliche Betäubung		
[ˌləʊkl ænəs'θetɪk]			

31 **use** [ju:s] Gebrauch
   video conferencing Videokonferenz
     ['vɪdiəʊ kɒnfərənsɪŋ]
   future ['fju:tʃə] Zukunft
   remote [rɪ'məʊt] fern, Fern-
   medical consultation medizinische Beratung
     [ˌmedɪkl kɒnsl'teɪʃn]
   take off [ˌteɪk 'ɒf] durchstarten, sich ver-
     breiten
   Scotland ['skɒtlənd] Schottland
   conduct [kən'dʌkt] durchführen
   experiment Versuch, Experiment
     [ɪk'sperɪmənt]
   medicine ['medsn] Medizin
   medical condition Leiden, Beschwerden
     [ˌmedɪkl kən'dɪʃn]
   trial ['traɪəl] Test
   whether ['weðə] ob
   face-to-face [ˌfeɪs tə 'feɪs] direkt, persönlich
   technology [tek'nɒlədʒi] Technik, Technologie
   present [prɪ'zent] zeigen, präsentieren
   life-size [ˌlaɪfsaɪz] lebensgroß
   image ['ɪmɪdʒ] Bild
   high-definition hochauflösend
     [ˌhaɪ defɪ'nɪʃn]
   as if [əz 'ɪf] als ob
   across [ə'krɒs] auf der anderen Seite
     von/des
   booth [bu:ð] Kabine
   device [dɪ'vaɪs] Gerät
   whole [həʊl] ganz
   setup ['setʌp] Aufbau, Anordnung,
     Einrichtung
   broadband ['brɔ:dbænd] Breitband
   network ['netwɜ:k] Netzwerk
   experience [ɪk'spɪəriəns] Erlebnis
   close [kləʊs] nahe, dicht
   volunteer [ˌvɒlən'tɪə] sich zur Verfügung stel-
     len
   stage [steɪdʒ] Phase, Abschnitt
   move sb [mu:v] *(Patienten)* verlegen
   safe [seɪf] sicher
   hands-on [ˌhændz 'ɒn] praktisch, direkt
   police station Polizeiwache
     [pə'li:s steɪʃn]
   succeed [sək'si:d] Erfolg haben, erfolgreich
     sein
   create [kri'eɪt] schaffen
   difficult ['dɪfɪkəlt] schwierig
   set up [ˌset 'ʌp] einrichten, aufbauen
   pilot trial ['paɪlət traɪəl] Pilotversuch, Pilotprojekt
   run sth [rʌn] etw leiten, führen
   ongoing ['ɒngəʊɪŋ] laufend, andauernd
   lesson ['lesn] Lehre, Lektion
   jigsaw ['dʒɪgsɔ:] Puzzle
   special ['speʃl] speziell, besonders
   summary ['sʌməri] Zusammenfassung

32 **pharmacy** ['fɑ:məsi] Apotheke
   fill a prescription ein Rezept dispensieren
     [ˌfɪl ə prɪ'skrɪpʃn]
   pharmacist ['fɑ:məsɪst] Apotheker/in
   warn [wɔ:n] warnen, darauf hinwei-
     sen
   over-the-counter frei verkäuflich
     [ˌəʊvə ðə 'kaʊntə]
   cough mixture Hustensaft
     ['kɒf mɪkstʃə]
   packet ['pækɪt] Packung
   chesty cough [ˌtʃesti 'kɒf] bronchialer Husten T
   dry [draɪ] trocken T
   come down with *(eine Krankheit)* bekom-
     [ˌkʌm 'daʊn wɪð] men, kriegen T
   cold [kəʊld] Erkältung T
   dosage ['dəʊsɪdʒ] Dosierung T
   teaspoonful ['ti:spu:nfʊl] Teelöffel T
   vaccine ['væksi:n] Impfstoff T
   suntan lotion Sonnenmilch
     [ˌsʌntæn 'ləʊʃn]
   contraceptive empfängnisverhütend,
     [ˌkɒntrə'septɪv] Empfängnisverhü-
     tungsmittel
   pill [pɪl] Pille
   cosmetics [kɒz'metɪks] Kosmetika
   painkiller ['peɪnkɪlə] Schmerzmittel
   sleeping tablet Schlaftablette
     ['sli:pɪŋ tæblət]
   laxative ['læksətɪv] Abführmittel
   anti-depressant Antidepressivum
     [ˌænti dɪ'presənt]
   cough sweet ['kɒf swi:t] Hustenbonbon
33 **capsule** ['kæpsju:l] Kapsel
   meal [mi:l] Mahlzeit, Essen
   effervescent tablet Brausetablette
     [efəˌvesnt 'tæblɪt]
   (shop) assistant Verkäufer/in
     ['ʃɒp əsɪstənt]
   customer ['kʌstəmə] Kunde/Kundin
   accept [ək'sept] akzeptieren
   urine sample Urinprobe
     ['jʊərɪn sɑ:mpl]
   cover ['kʌvə] *(Kosten)* decken
   physiotherapy Physiotherapie
     [ˌfi:ziəʊ'θerəpi]
   side effect ['saɪd ɪfekt] Nebenwirkung
   medication [ˌmedɪ'keɪʃn] Medikamente, Medika-
     tion
   drop [drɒp] Tropfen
   sugared pill [ˌʃʊgəd 'pɪl] Dragee
34 **instruction(s)** Anleitung
     [ɪn'strʌkʃnz]
   leave out [ˌli:v 'aʊt] weglassen
   unless [ən'les] wenn nicht

otherwise [ˈʌðəwaɪz] — anders
empty [ˈempti] — leer
dissolve [dɪˈzɒlv] — auflösen
allow to dissolve — zergehen lassen
[əˌlaʊ tə dɪˈzɒlv]
minority [maɪˈnɒrəti] — Minderzahl
case [keɪs] — Fall
drowsiness [ˈdraʊzinəs] — Schläfrigkeit
nausea [ˈnɔːziə] — Übelkeit
stomach complaints — Magenbeschwerden
[ˈstʌmək kəmpleɪnts]
blurred vision — verschwommenes Sehen
[ˌblɜːd ˈvɪʒn]

35 unfortunately — leider
[ʌnˈfɔːtʃənətli]
mistake [mɪˈsteɪk] — Fehler
head office [ˌhed ˈɒfɪs] — Zentrale, Hauptsitz
compare [kəmˈpeə] — vergleichen
shipment [ˈʃɪpmənt] — Sendung, Lieferung
item [ˈaɪtəm] — Artikel
bottle [ˈbɒtl] — Flasche
saline [ˈseɪlaɪn] — Salz-
infusion [ɪnˈfjuːʒn] — Infusion
saline infusion — Kochsalzlösung
[ˌseɪlaɪn ɪnˈfjuːʒn]
pump [pʌmp] — Pumpe
dose [dəʊs] — Dosis
disposable [dɪˈspəʊzəbl] — Einweg-
tin [tɪn] — Dose
antiseptic [ˌænti'septɪk] — antiseptisch
ointment [ˈɔɪntmənt] — Salbe, Wundsalbe
deliver [dɪˈlɪvə] — liefern T
several [ˈsevrəl] — einige, mehrere T
Hold on. [ˌhəʊld ˈɒn] — Einen Moment. T
call up [ˌkɔːl ˈʌp] — aufrufen T
order [ˈɔːdə] — Bestellung T
amount [əˈmaʊnt] — Menge T
serious [ˈsɪəriəs] — schwer, ernst T
minor [ˈmaɪnə] — klein, gering T
My goodness. — Meine Güte! T
[ˌmaɪ ˈɡʊdnəs]
till [tɪl] — bis T
express [ɪkˈspres] — per Eilbote T
pick up [ˌpɪk ˈʌp] — abholen T
Fair enough. [ˌfeər ɪˈnʌf] — Na gut. Einverstanden. T
as long as [əz ˈlɒŋ əz] — solange T
arrive [əˈraɪv] — ankommen, eintreffen T
promise [ˈprɒmɪs] — versprechen T
mix-up [ˈmɪks ʌp] — Durcheinander, Verwechslung T
serve sb [sɜːv] — jdn bedienen

36 map [mæp] — Karte, Plan
place [pleɪs] — Platz, Ort
optician [ɒpˈtɪʃn] — Optiker
bus station [ˈbʌs steɪʃn] — Busbahnhof

corner [ˈkɔːnə] — Ecke
car park [ˈkɑː pɑːk] — Parkplatz
pedestrian subway — Fußgängerunterführung
[pɪˌdestriən ˈsʌbweɪ]
sketch [sketʃ] — Skizze
starting point — Ausgangspunkt
[ˈstɑːtɪŋ pɔɪnt]
finishing point — Ziel
[ˈfɪnɪʃɪŋ pɔɪnt]
until [ənˈtɪl] — bis
on foot [ɒn ˈfʊt] — zu Fuß T
exercise [ˈeksəsaɪz] — Bewegung, Sport T
crossroads [ˈkrɒsrəʊdz] — Kreuzung T
cross [krɒs] — überqueren T
reach [riːtʃ] — erreichen T

37 sound [saʊnd] — klingen T
arrange [əˈreɪndʒ] — arrangieren, vereinbaren
mobile phone — Handy
[ˌməʊbaɪl ˈfəʊn]
join sb [dʒɔɪn] — sich jdm anschließen
stand [stænd] — stehen
fancy sth [ˈfænsi] — Lust auf etw haben
meet (sb) [miːt] — sich (mit jdm) treffen
bargain [ˈbɑːɡɪn] — Schnäppchen
delicious [dɪˈlɪʃəs] — delikat, lecker
cheap [tʃiːp] — billig, preiswert
unusual [ʌnˈjuːʒuəl] — ungewöhnlich, außergewöhnlich
diner [ˈdaɪnə] — Imbissstube, Lokal
cart [kɑːt] — Karren
candy [ˈkændi] — Süßigkeiten
weather [ˈweðə] — Wetter
sunny [ˈsʌni] — sonnig
pleasant [ˈpleznt] — angenehm

38 sexual [ˈsekʃuəl] — sexuell
transmit [trænsˈmɪt] — übertragen
rise [raɪz] — Anstieg, Zunahme
refer to sth [rɪˈfɜː tə] — sich auf etw beziehen
gone [gɒn] — weg, verschwunden
forget [fəˈget] — vergessen
belief [bɪˈliːf] — Glaube, Überzeugung
among [əˈmʌŋ] — unter
virus [ˈvaɪrəs] — Virus
cure [kjʊə] — heilen
level [ˈlevl] — hier: Rate, Quote
report [rɪˈpɔːt] — Bericht
cure [kjʊə] — Heilmittel; Heilung, Therapie
fail to do sth [feɪl] — versäumen, etw zu tun
adequate [ˈædɪkwət] — angemessen
precaution [prɪˈkɔːʃn] — Vorkehrung, Vorsichtsmaßnahme
prevent [prɪˈvent] — verhüten, verhindern
spread [spred] — Ausbreitung
trust [trʌst] — Stiftung
charity [ˈtʃærəti] — Wohlfahrtsorganisation

	sufferer [ˈsʌfərə]	Erkrankte/r, Patient/in	
	rise [raɪz]	ansteigen	
	research [rɪˈsɜːtʃ]	Forschung, Untersuchungen	
	suggest [səˈdʒest]	hinweisen auf, hindeuten auf	
	widespread [ˈwaɪdspred]	weit verbreitet	
	ignorance [ˈɪɡnərəns]	Unkenntnis, Unwissen	
	especially [ɪˈspeʃəli]	besonders	
	poll [pəʊl]	Umfrage	
	find [faɪnd]	herausfinden, feststellen	
	aged [eɪdʒd]	im Alter von	
	mistakenly [mɪˈsteɪkənli]	fälschlich	
	health protection [ˈhelθ prətekʃn]	Gesundheitsschutz, -vorsorge	
	agency [ˈeɪdʒənsi]	Agentur, Behörde	
	diagnosis, diagnoses [ˌdaɪəɡˈnəʊsɪs, daɪəɡˈnəʊsiːz]	Diagnose, Diagnosen	
	largely [ˈlɑːdʒli]	hauptsächlich, vor allem	
	gay [ɡeɪ]	schwul	
	continually [kənˈtɪnjuəli]	stetig, kontinuierlich	
	since [sɪns]	seit	
	increase [ˈɪŋkriːs]	Steigerung	
	in recent years [ɪn ˈriːsnt jɪəz]	in den letzten Jahren	
	be due to sth [bi ˈdjuː tə]	auf etw zurückzuführen sein	
	head [hed]	Chef/in	
	rate [reɪt]	Quote, Rate	
	active [ˈæktɪv]	aktiv	
	content [kənˈtent]	Inhalt	
	public [ˈpʌblɪk]	öffentlich	
	grow [ɡrəʊ]	wachsen, zunehmen, steigen	
	experience [ɪkˈspɪəriəns]	erleben, erfahren	
	overall [ˌəʊvərˈɔːl]	Gesamt-	

39 **examination couch** [ɪɡˌzæmɪˈneɪʃn kaʊtʃ] — Untersuchungsliege, Behandlungsliege
sick [sɪk] — krank
prepare [prɪˈpeə] — (sich) vorbereiten
presentation [ˌpreznˈteɪʃn] — Präsentation
poem [ˈpəʊɪm] — Gedicht
broad [brɔːd] — breit
rump [rʌmp] — Rumpf
gentle [ˈdʒentl] — sanft
pull [pʊl] — ziehen
crisis, crises [ˈkraɪsɪs, ˈkraɪsiːz] — Krise, Krisen

Unit 6

40 **need** [niːd] — Bedürfnis
pelvic examination [ˌpelvɪk ɪɡzæmɪˈneɪʃn] — gynäkologische Untersuchung
prescription medication [prɪˈskrɪpʃn medɪkeɪʃn] — verschreibungspflichtige Medikamente

smallpox [ˈsmɔːlpɒks] — Pocken
physical [ˈfɪzɪkl] — körperlich
mental [ˈmentl] — geistig
suggestion [səˈdʒestʃən] — Vorschlag
hearing aid [ˈhɪərɪŋ eɪd] — Hörgerät
wheelchair [ˈwiːltʃeə] — Rollstuhl
pushchair [ˈpʊʃtʃeə] — Buggy (Kinderwagen)
Chinese [tʃaɪˈniːz] — chinesisch
undress [ˌʌnˈdres] — sich ausziehen
explanation [ˌekspləˈneɪʃn] — Erklärung, Erläuterung
disabled [dɪsˈeɪbld] — behindert
partially [ˈpɑːʃəli] — teilweise, zum Teil
scary [ˈskeəri] — unheimlich T
renew [rɪˈnjuː] — erneuern T
normally [ˈnɔːməli] — normalerweise T
phone in [ˌfəʊn ˈɪn] — anrufen T
beach [biːtʃ] — Strand T
awful [ˈɔːfl] — schrecklich, fürchterlich T
germ [dʒɜːm] — Keim, Bakterie T
spread [spred] — verbreiten T

41 **traditional** [trəˈdɪʃnəl] — traditionell
emigrant [ˈemɪɡrənt] — Auswanderer
businessman [ˈbɪznəsmən] — Geschäftsmann
violinist [ˌvaɪəˈlɪnɪst] — Geiger/in
rate [reɪt] — einstufen
tense [tens] — angespannt
worried [ˈwʌrid] — besorgt, beunruhigt
dental [ˈdentl] — Zahn-
job interview [ˈdʒɒb ɪntəvjuː] — Vorstellungsgespräch
express [ɪkˈspres] — ausdrücken
be scared of sth [bi ˈskeəd əv] — vor etw Angst haben
feel uncomfortable [ˌfiːl ʌnˈkʌmftəbl] — sich unwohl fühlen
anxiety [æŋˈzaɪəti] — Angst, Sorge
paragraph [ˈpærəɡrɑːf] — (Text:) Absatz
fear [fɪə] — Furcht, Angst
death [deθ] — Tod
poor [pʊə] — schlecht, dürftig

42 **be afraid of sth** [bi əˈfreɪd əv] — vor etw Angst haben
atmosphere [ˈætməsfɪə] — Atmosphäre, Stimmung
smell (of sth) [smel] — (nach etw) riechen
cause [kɔːz] — Ursache, Grund
fact [fækt] — Tatsache
cancer [ˈkænsə] — Krebs
life-threatening [ˈlaɪf θretnɪŋ] — lebensbedrohlich
ill [ɪl] — krank
coldness [ˈkəʊldnəs] — Kälte
scare sb [skeə] — jdm Angst einjagen, jdn erschrecken

friendly ['frendli]	freundlich	
sheet [ʃiːt]	Blatt (Papier)	
associate sb with sth	jdn mit etw in Verbin-	
[ə'səʊʃieɪt wɪð]	dung bringen	
involve [ɪn'vɒlv]	mit sich bringen	
helpless ['helpləs]	hilflos	
control [kən'trəʊl]	Kontrolle	
would rather not hear	würden die Wahrheit	
the truth [wʊd ˌrɑːðə	lieber nicht erfahren	
nɒt ˌhɪə ðə 'truːθ]		
risk [rɪsk]	Risiko	
catch sth [kætʃ]	sich mit etw anstecken	
unfriendly [ʌn'frendli]	unfreundlich	
common ['kɒmən]	üblich, verbreitet	

43 **discomfort** [dɪs'kʌmfət] Unbehagen, Schmerz
emotion [ɪ'məʊʃn] Gefühl, Emotion
helplessness ['helpləsnəs] Hilflosigkeit
smelly ['smeli] stinkend
scare [skeə] Schrecken
risky ['rɪski] riskant
carefully ['keəfəli] sorgfältig, genau
be faced with sb mit jdm konfrontiert
[bi 'feɪst wɪð] werden
sense [sens] Sinn
bronchoscope Bronchoskop
['brɒŋkəʊskəʊp]
artery ['ɑːtəri] Arterie
artery forceps Arterienklemme
['ɑːtəri fɔːseps]
speculum ['spekjʊləm] Spekulum

44 **advice** [əd'vaɪs] (guter) Rat, Ratschlag
useful ['juːsfl] nützlich, geeignet
relaxing [rɪ'læksɪŋ] entspannend
watch TV [ˌwɒtʃ tiː'viː] fernsehen
during ['djʊərɪŋ] während
foot spa ['fʊt spɑː] Fußbad
massage ['mæsɑːʒ] massieren
candle ['kændl] Kerze
nowadays ['naʊədeɪz] heutzutage
improvement Verbesserung
[ɪm'pruːvmənt]
relaxed [rɪ'lækst] locker, entspannt
invasive [ɪn'veɪsɪv] invasiv
spend [spend] *(Zeit)* verbringen
painless ['peɪnləs] schmerzlos T
possible ['pɒsəbl] möglich T
expect [ɪk'spekt] erwarten T
benefit ['benɪfɪt] Nutzen, Vorteil T
suppose [sə'pəʊz] annehmen, glauben T
mean [miːn] bedeuten, heißen T
progress ['prəʊgres] Fortschritt T
trust sb [trʌst] jdm vertrauen T
properly ['prɒpəli] richtig, ordentlich T
rushed [rʌʃt] gehetzt T
burn a candle eine Kerze verwenden,
[ˌbɜːn ə 'kændl] brennen lassen T

massage ['mæsɑːʒ]	Massage T	
relieve [rɪ'liːv]	lindern, abbauen T	
offer ['ɒfə]	anbieten, bieten	
reassurance	Beruhigung	
[ˌriːə'ʃʊərəns]		

45 **lie around** [ˌlaɪ ə'raʊnd] herumliegen

46 **procedure** [prə'siːdʒə] Eingriff
perfectly ['pɜːfɪktli] völlig
breast [brest] Brust T
lie down [ˌlaɪ 'daʊn] sich hinlegen T
cell [sel] Zelle T
cervix ['sɜːvɪks] Gebärmutterhals T
wooden stick Holzstab T
[ˌwʊdn 'stɪk]
brush [brʌʃ] Bürste, Pinsel T
absolutely ['æbsəluːtli] völlig, absolut, ganz T
internal [ɪn'tɜːnl] innere/r/s T
right away [raɪt ə'weɪ] sofort T
in detail [ɪn 'diːteɪl] im einzelnen T
vaccination Impfung
[ˌvæksɪ'neɪʃn]
make sth up [ˌmeɪk 'ʌp] sich etw ausdenken, etw
erfinden

47 **carer** ['keərə] Betreuer/in, Pfleger/in
relationship [rɪ'leɪʃnʃɪp] Verhältnis, Beziehung
train (as) [treɪn əz] eine Ausbildung machen
(zum)
care [keə] Betreuung, Pflege
health and social care Gesundheitswesen und
[ˌhelθ ənd 'səʊʃl keə] Sozialfürsorge
avoid [ə'vɔɪd] vermeiden
talk [tɔːk] Vortrag
honest ['ɒnɪst] ehrlich, aufrichtig
client ['klaɪənt] Klient/in, Kunde/Kundin
look after sb [ˌlʊk 'ɑːftə] sich um jdn kümmern
patient ['peɪʃnt] geduldig
success [sək'ses] Erfolg T
rely on sth [rɪ'laɪ ɒn] auf etw angewiesen
sein T
task [tɑːsk] Aufgabe T
human ['hjuːmən] menschlich T
warmth [wɔːmθ] Wärme T
understanding verständnisvoll T
[ˌʌndə'stændɪŋ]
angry ['æŋgri] ungehalten, wütend T
frustrated [frʌ'streɪtɪd] frustriert T
essential [ɪ'senʃl] wesentlich, notwendig T
react [ri'ækt] reagieren T
ill-tempered [ˌɪl'tempəd] griesgrämig, verärgert T
lonely ['ləʊnli] einsam T
weakness ['wiːknəs] Schwäche T
lazy ['leɪzi] faul T
reduce [rɪ'djuːs] verringern T
self-respect Selbstachtung T
[ˌself rɪ'spekt]

self-esteem [ˌself ɪ'sti:m]	Selbstwertgefühl T	
rush around [ˌrʌʃ ə'raʊnd]	umherhetzen T	
actually ['æktʃuəli]	wirklich, tatsächlich T	
honesty ['ɒnəsti]	Ehrlichkeit, Aufrichtig-keit T	
apologize [ə'pɒlədʒaɪz]	sich entschuldigen T	
trust [trʌst]	Vertrauen T	
take care of sb [teɪk 'keər əv]	auf jdn aufpassen, sich um jdn kümmern T	
take time off [teɪk ˌtaɪm 'ɒf]	sich freinehmen, sich Zeit nehmen T	
enjoy [ɪn'dʒɔɪ]	genießen, gern tun T	
make sure [ˌmeɪk 'ʃʊə]	dafür sorgen T	
manager ['mænɪdʒə]	Geschäftsführer/in T	
outside ['aʊtsaɪd]	außerhalb T	
occur [ə'kɜ:]	auftreten	
solve [sɒlv]	lösen	
disability [ˌdɪsə'bɪləti]	Behinderung	
support organization [sə'pɔ:t ɔ:gənaɪzeɪʃn]	Hilfsorganisation	
the elderly [ði 'eldəli]	ältere Menschen, Senio-ren	
rest home ['rest həʊm]	Seniorenheim	
database ['deɪtəbeɪs]	Datenbank	
provider [prə'vaɪdə]	Anbieter	
retirement [rɪ'taɪəmənt]	Ruhestand	
issue ['ɪʃu:]	Frage, Problem	

Unit 7

48	**nutrition** [nju'trɪʃn]	Ernährung
	healthy ['helθi]	gesund
	decide [dɪ'saɪd]	entscheiden
	recent ['ri:snt]	aktuell, jüngere/r/s, letzte/r/s
	scientific [ˌsaɪən'tɪfɪk]	wissenschaftlich
	study ['stʌdi]	Untersuchung, Studie
	obese [əʊ'bi:s]	fettleibig
	diet ['daɪət]	Ernährung, Kost
	be badly behaved [bi ˌbædli bɪ'heɪvd]	sich schlecht benehmen, unartig sein
	according to [ə'kɔ:dɪŋ tə]	laut, nach, gemäß
	expert ['ekspɜ:t]	Experte/-in, Fachmann/-frau
	contain [kən'teɪn]	enthalten
	plum [plʌm]	Pflaume
	reckon ['rekən]	schätzen
	percentage [pə'sentɪdʒ]	Anteil, Prozentsatz
	calorie ['kæləri]	Kalorie
	intake ['ɪnteɪk]	Zufuhr
	carbohydrates [ˌkɑːbəʊ'haɪdreɪts]	Kohlenhydrate
49	**chart** [tʃɑ:t]	Grafik
	fat [fæt]	Fett
	oil [ɔɪl]	Öl
	meat [mi:t]	Fleisch
	cold cut [ˌkəʊld 'kʌt]	Aufschnitt

	dairy products ['deəri prɒdʌkts]	Molkereiprodukte, Milchprodukte
	cereal ['sɪəriəl]	Getreide, Getreide-flocken
	cream [kri:m]	Sahne
	biscuit ['bɪskɪt]	Keks
	bread roll [ˌbred 'rəʊl]	Brötchen
	juice [dʒu:s]	Saft
	salmon ['sæmən]	Lachs
	chicken ['tʃɪkɪn]	Huhn
	sausage ['sɒsɪdʒ]	(Brat-)Wurst
	onion ['ʌnjən]	Zwiebel
	maple syrup [ˌmeɪpl 'sɪrəp]	Ahornsirup
	consume [kən'sju:m]	verzehren
	high-fibre ['haɪfaɪbə]	ballaststoffreich
	pregnancy ['pregnənsi]	Schwangerschaft
	harmful ['hɑ:mfl]	schädlich
	coconut ['kəʊkənʌt]	Kokosnuss
	olive ['ɒlɪv]	Olive
	rapeseed (BE), **canola** (AE) ['reɪpsi:d, kə'nəʊlə]	Raps
	unsweetened [ˌʌn'swi:tnd]	ungesüßt
	sweeten ['swi:tn]	süßen
	recommend [ˌrekə'mend]	empfehlen T
	folic acid [ˌfəʊlɪk 'æsɪd]	Folsäure T
	cabbage ['kæbɪdʒ]	Kohl T
	spinach ['spɪnɪtʃ]	Spinat T
	harm [hɑ:m]	schädigen, schaden T
	foetus ['fi:təs]	Fötus T
	smoker ['sməʊkə]	Raucher/in T
	beef [bi:f]	Rind(fleisch) T
	pork [pɔ:k]	Schwein(efleisch) T
	palm oil ['pɑ:m ɔɪl]	Palmöl T
	limit ['lɪmɪt]	begrenzen, beschrän-ken T
	anything in particular [ˌeniθɪŋ ɪn pə'tɪkjələ]	etwas Besonderes T
	have a sweet tooth [həv ə ˌswi:t 'tu:θ]	eine Vorliebe für Süßes haben T
	naturally ['nætʃrəli]	von Natur aus T
50	**cholesterol** [kə'lestərɒl]	Cholesterin
	fibre ['faɪbə]	Ballaststoffe
	below [bɪ'ləʊ]	unterhalb
	grain [greɪn]	Korn
	pass through [ˌpɑ:s 'θru:]	hindurchgehen
	substance ['sʌbstəns]	Stoff, Substanz
	skimmed milk [ˌskɪmd 'mɪlk]	entrahmte/fettarme Milch
	full fat milk [ˌfʊl fæt 'mɪlk]	Vollmilch
	saturated ['sætʃəreɪtɪd]	gesättigt
	dangerous ['deɪndʒərəs]	gefährlich
	level ['levl]	Spiegel
	cholesterol level [kə'lestərol levl]	Cholesterinspiegel

jar [dʒɑː] — Glas

prepare [prɪ'peə] — (Essen) kochen, zubereiten

rich (in) ['rɪtʃ ɪn] — reich (an)

vegetable oil ['vedʒtəbl ɔɪl] — Pflanzenöl

high in fibre [ˌhaɪ ɪn 'faɪbə] — ballaststoffreich

honey ['hʌni] — Honig

condition [kən'dɪʃn] — Zustand

improve [ɪm'pruːv] — (sich) bessern, verbessern

51 wordfield ['wɜːdfiːld] — Wortfeld

produce [prə'djuːs] — herstellen, erstellen

diabetes [ˌdaɪə'biːtiːz] — Diabetes

commonly ['kɒmənli] — häufig, gewöhnlich

contagious [kən'teɪdʒəs] — ansteckend

genetic [dʒə'netɪk] — genetisch, erblich

environmental [ɪnˌvaɪrən'mentl] — Umwelt-

develop [dɪ'veləp] — entwickeln

type [taɪp] — Typ

equally ['iːkwəli] — gleich, gleichermaßen

lead [liːd] — führen

insulin ['ɪnsjʊlɪn] — Insulin

coach [kəʊtʃ] — Reisebus

gold medal [ˌgəʊld 'medl] — Goldmedaille

rower ['rəʊə] — Ruderer/-in

do exercise [du: 'eksəsaɪz] — sich bewegen, Sport treiben

lifestyle ['laɪfstaɪl] — Lebensweise, Lebensführung

advise [əd'vaɪz] — raten, beraten

flu jab ['fluː dʒæb] — Grippeimpfung

change [tʃeɪndʒ] — (sich) verändern, (sich) ändern

blood glucose control [ˌblʌd 'gluːkəʊz kəntrəʊl] — Blutzuckerregulation

put sb at risk [ˌpʊt ət 'rɪsk] — jdn einem Risiko aussetzen

blood glucose level [ˌblʌd 'gluːkəʊz levl] — Blutzuckerspiegel

sugary ['ʃʊgəri] — süß, zuckerhaltig

rest [rest] — Rest

confectionery foods [kənˌfekʃnəri 'fuːdz] — Süßwaren, Konditoreierzeugnisse

lose weight [ˌluːz 'weɪt] — abnehmen

52 the odd one out [ði ˌɒd wʌn 'aʊt] — etwas, das nicht dazugehört

fit [fɪt] — passen

danger ['deɪndʒə] — Gefahr

control [kən'trəʊl] — kontrollieren, regulieren

still [stɪl] — trotzdem, dennoch

day-to-day [ˌdeɪ tə 'deɪ] — täglich T

change [tʃeɪndʒ] — Änderung, Veränderung T

self-care [ˌself 'keə] — Eigenfürsorge T

monitor ['mɒnɪtə] — überwachen T

crazy ['kreɪzi] — verrückt T

chest infection ['tʃest ɪnfekʃn] — Lungeninfekt T

progressive [prə'gresɪv] — fortschreitend, progressiv T

damage ['dæmɪdʒ] — Schaden, Schäden T

nerve [nɜːv] — Nerv T

53 chef [ʃef] — Koch/Köchin

fight [faɪt] — kämpfen

school dinner ['skuːl dɪnə] — Schulessen

guidelines ['gaɪdlaɪnz] — Richtlinien

mark [mɑːk] — markieren

victory ['vɪktəri] — Sieg

latest ['leɪtɪst] — letzte/r/s, jüngste/r/s

fight [faɪt] — Kampf

introduce [ˌɪntrə'djuːs] — einführen

habit ['hæbɪt] — Gewohnheit

feed [fiːd] — ernähren, verpflegen

campaign [kæm'peɪn] — Kampagne, Aktion

because of [bɪ'kɒz əv] — wegen

serve [sɜːv] — servieren

TV programme [ˌtiː'viː prəʊgræm] — Fernsehsendung

rather than ['rɑːðə ðən] — statt

chips [tʃɪps] — Pommes frites

carbonated ['kɑːbəneɪtɪd] — kohlensäurehaltig

TV show [ˌtiː 'viː ʃəʊ] — Fernsehsendung

viewer ['vjuːə] — Zuschauer/in

report [rɪ'pɔːt] — berichten

just [dʒʌst] — nur, gerade, bloß

government ['gʌvənmənt] — Regierung

despite [dɪ'spaɪt] — trotz

popularity [ˌpɒpju'lærəti] — Beliebtheit

award-winning [ə'wɔːd wɪnɪŋ] — preisgekrönt

introduction [ˌɪntrə'dʌkʃn] — Einführung

far from over [ˌfɑː frəm 'əʊvə] — noch lange nicht vorbei

drop [drɒp] — Rückgang

black market [ˌblæk 'mɑːkɪt] — Schwarzmarkt

non-nutritional foods [ˌnɒn njuːtrɪʃnəl 'fuːdz] — Lebensmittel ohne Nährwert

van [væn] — Lieferwagen

school gates ['skuːl geɪts] — Schultor

destroy [dɪ'strɔɪ] — zerstören

pros and cons [ˌprəʊz ənd 'kɒnz] — Pro und Contra

bubble ['bʌbl] — (Luft-)Blase

54	**deal with sth** ['di:l wɪð]	mit etw umgehen, mit etw fertig werden, mit etw zurecht kommen
	phrase [freɪz]	Redewendung, Ausdruck
	assume the worst [ə,sju:m ðə 'wɜ:st]	das Schlimmste befürchten
	worry about sth ['wʌri əbaʊt]	sich um etw Sorgen machen
	sensation [sen'seɪʃn]	Gefühl, Empfindung
	strange [streɪndʒ]	seltsam T
	pins and needles [,pɪnz ənd 'ni:dlz]	Kribbeln T
	kind of ['kaɪnd əv]	irgendwie T
	weird [wɪəd]	seltsam, unheimlich T
	depressed [dɪ'prest]	niedergeschlagen, deprimiert T
	vision ['vɪʒn]	Sehen, Sehkraft T
	tingling ['tɪŋglɪŋ]	Kribbeln T
	bladder ['blædə]	Blase T
	bowel ['baʊəl]	Darm T
	the other day [ði ,ʌðə 'deɪ]	neulich T
	analysis, analyses [ə'næləsɪs, ə'næləsi:z]	Analyse, Analysen T
	remove [rɪ'mu:v]	(Kleidung) ausziehen T
55	**bracket** ['brækɪt]	Klammer
	hurry up [,hʌri 'ʌp]	sich beeilen
	neurologist [njʊə'rɒlədʒɪst]	Neurologe/-in
	short of breath [,ʃɔːt əv 'breθ]	außer Atem
	stone [stəʊn]	Stein
	affect [ə'fekt]	betreffen, beeinträchtigen
	bend [bend]	beugen
	whiplash ['wɪplæʃ]	Schleudertrauma
	car crash ['kɑ: kræʃ]	Autounfall
	resonance ['rezənəns]	Resonanz
	imaging ['ɪmɪdʒɪŋ]	Bildgebung
	cutaway ['kʌtəweɪ]	Schnittbild, Schnittansicht
	radio frequency [,reɪdiəʊ 'fri:kwənsi]	Funkwellenlänge
	gradient coils [,greɪdiənt 'kɔɪlz]	Neigungsspulen
56	**Nice to meet you.** [,naɪs tə 'mi:t ju]	Schön, Sie kennenzulernen.
	fill in [,fɪl 'ɪn]	*(Formular)* ausfüllen
	gown [gaʊn]	Kittel
	watch [wɒtʃ]	Armbanduhr
	jewellery ['dʒu:əlri]	Schmuck
	bra [brɑ:]	BH
	clasp [klɑ:sp]	Verschluss, Schließe
	lie back [,laɪ 'bæk]	sich auf den Rücken legen

	move [mu:v]	bewegen
	noisy ['nɔɪzi]	laut
	earplug ['ɪəplʌg]	Ohrstöpsel
	pad [pæd]	Polster, Kissen
	blanket ['blæŋkɪt]	Decke
	loud [laʊd]	laut
	bang [bæŋ]	knallen
	noise [nɔɪz]	Geräusch
	last [lɑ:st]	dauern
	Are you comfortable? [,ɑ: ju: 'kʌmftəbl]	*hier:* Liegen Sie bequem?
	get started [,get 'stɑːtɪd]	anfangen
	multiple sclerosis [,mʌltɪpl sklə'rəʊsɪs]	Multiple Sklerose
	attack [ə'tæk]	angreifen, befallen
	expensive [ɪk'spensɪv]	teuer
57	**known** [nəʊn]	bekannt
	perhaps [pə'hæps]	vielleicht
	immune system [ɪ'mju:n sɪstəm]	Immunsystem
	central ['sentrəl]	zentral
	nervous system [,nɜ:vəs 'sɪstəm]	Nervensystem
	transfer ['trænsfɜ:]	Übermittlung
	message ['mesɪdʒ]	Botschaft, Nachricht
	occur [ə'kɜ:]	vorkommen
	currently ['kʌrəntli]	derzeit, zurzeit, momentan
	focus on sth ['fəʊkəs ɒn]	sich auf etw konzentrieren
	ease [i:z]	lindern
	horizon [hə'raɪzn]	Horizont
	researcher [rɪ'sɜ:tʃə]	Forscher/in, Wissenschaftler/in
	possibly ['pɒsəbli]	möglicherweise
	development [dɪ'veləpmənt]	Entwicklung
	be able to [bi 'eɪbl tə]	in der Lage sein
	mouse, mice [maʊs, maɪs]	Maus, Mäuse
	galanin [gɑ:'lʌnɪn]	Galanin
	nerve cell ['nɜ:v sel]	Nervenzelle
	find [faɪnd]	entdecken, herausfinden
	protein ['prəʊti:n]	Protein
	injure ['ɪndʒə]	verletzen
	increase [ɪn'kri:s]	ansteigen
	dramatically [drə'mætɪkli]	drastisch
	cell death ['sel deθ]	Zelltod
	prove [pru:v]	beweisen, nachweisen
	in contrast [ɪn 'kɒntrɑːst]	im Gegensatz dazu, dagegen
	slow (down) [,sləʊ 'daʊn]	verlangsamen
	progress ['prəʊgres]	Verlauf
	race [reɪs]	Rasse

59	progress [prə'gres]	verlaufen
	subtype ['sʌbtaɪp]	Subtyp, Untertyp
	Primary-progressive MS	Primär-progrediente MS
	[ˌpraɪməri prə'gresɪv]	
	Secondary-progressive	Sekundär-progrediente
	MS [ˌsekəndri prə'gresɪv]	MS
	Relapsing-remitting MS	Schubförmig-remittie-
	[rɪˌlæpsɪŋ rɪ'mɪtɪŋ]	rende MS
	Progressive-relapsing	Schubförmig-progre-
	MS [prəˌgresɪv rɪ'læpsɪŋ]	diente MS
	stage [steɪdʒ]	Stadium T
	definite ['defɪnət]	sicher, bestimmt, defini-
		tiv T
	rule sth out [ˌru:l 'aʊt]	etw ausschließen T
	separate ['seprət]	einzeln, getrennt T
	attack [ə'tæk]	Anfall, Attacke T
	steady ['stedi]	stetig, gleichmäßig T
	decline [dɪ'klaɪn]	Rückgang T
	period ['pɪəriəd]	Zeitraum, Zeitab-
		schnitt T
	predict [prɪ'dɪkt]	voraussagen T
	future ['fju:tʃə]	zukünftig T
	course [kɔ:s]	Verlauf T
	relapse [rɪ'læps]	Schub T
	remission [rɪ'mɪʃn]	Abklingen, Remission T
	frequent ['fri:kwənt]	häufig T
	grow worse [ˌgrəʊ 'wɜ:s]	sich verschlimmern T
	uncommon [ʌn'kɒmən]	selten, ungewöhnlich T
	interval ['ɪntəvl]	Abstand T
60	dormant ['dɔ:mənt]	ruhend, nicht aktiv
	past [pɑ:st]	Vergangenheit
	recognized ['rekəgnaɪzd]	anerkannt
	appear [ə'pɪə]	auftreten
	strike [straɪk]	zuschlagen
	South African	südafrikanisch, aus
	[saʊθ 'æfrɪkən]	Südafrika
	act [ækt]	spielen
	technician [tek'nɪʃn]	Techniker/in
	hand over [ˌhænd 'əʊvə]	übergeben
61	**case study** ['keɪs stʌdi]	Fallstudie
	fit [fɪt]	fit, in Form
	career [kə'rɪə]	Beruf, Laufbahn,
		Karriere
	long-distance runner	Langstreckenläufer/in
	[ˌlɒŋ'dɪstəns rʌnə]	
	wake up [ˌweɪk 'ʌp]	aufwachen
	numb [nʌm]	(Gefühl:) taub
	carry on [ˌkæri 'ɒn]	weitermachen
	undergo [ˌʌndə'gəʊ]	sich unterziehen, durch-
		machen
	lumbar puncture	Lumbalpunktion
	[ˌlʌmbə 'pʌŋktʃə]	
	numbness ['nʌmnəs]	Taubheit
	continue to do sth	etw weiterhin tun
	[kən'tɪnju:]	
	research sth [rɪ'sɜ:tʃ]	sich über etw erkundigen

	fight back [ˌfaɪt 'bæk]	sich wehren
	varied ['veərid]	verschieden(artig),
		abwechslungsreich
	constant ['kɒnstənt]	ständig
	get on (with sth)	(mit etw) vorankommen
	[ˌget 'ɒn wɪð]	
	arise [ə'raɪz]	auftreten, auftauchen
	outlook ['aʊtlʊk]	Einstellung
	what life has to throw	etwa: was das Leben
	at sb [wɒt ˌlaɪf həz tə	einem zu bieten hat
	'θrəʊ ət]	
	go by [ˌgəʊ 'baɪ]	vorübergehen, vergehen
	alter ['ɔ:ltə]	verändern
	open ['əʊpən]	öffnen
	allow [ə'laʊ]	gestatten, erlauben
	although [ɔ:l'ðəʊ]	obwohl
	retire [rɪ'taɪə]	sich zur Ruhe setzen
	secretary ['sekrətri]	Sekretär/in
	society [sə'saɪəti]	Gesellschaft
	support centre	Hilfszentrum
	[sə'pɔ:t sentə]	
	keep sb active	jdn auf Trab halten
	[ˌki:p 'æktɪv]	
	supportive [sə'pɔ:tɪv]	verständnisvoll
	author ['ɔ:θə]	Autor/in, Verfasser/in
	final line [ˌfaɪnl 'laɪn]	letzte Zeile

Unit 9

62	disorder [dɪs'ɔ:də]	Störung
	eating disorder	Essstörung
	[ˌi:tɪŋ dɪs'ɔ:də]	
	advice column	(Zeitschrift:) Kummer-
	[əd'vaɪs kɒləm]	kasten
	thin [θɪn]	dünn
	mental illness	psychische Erkrankung
	[ˌmentl 'ɪlnəs]	
	obsession [əb'seʃn]	Besessenheit, Wahn,
		Zwang
	looks [lʊks]	Aussehen
	weight [weɪt]	Gewicht
	sickness ['sɪknəs]	Übelkeit
	stupid ['stju:pɪd]	töricht, doof
	obesity [əʊ'bi:səti]	Fettleibigkeit
	mass [mæs]	Masse
	divided by [dɪ'vaɪdɪd baɪ]	geteilt durch
	square [skweə]	Quadrat
	height [haɪt]	Körpergröße
	anorexia [ˌænə'reksiə]	Anorexie
	bulimia [bu:'lɪmiə]	Bulimie
	overeating [ˌəʊvər'i:tɪŋ]	übermäßiges Essen
	irregular [ɪ'regjələ]	unregelmäßig
	low [ləʊ]	niedrig
	circulation [ˌsɜ:kjə'leɪʃn]	Kreislauf, Zirkulation
	purging (controlled	kontrolliertes Erbrechen
	vomiting) ['pɜ:dʒɪŋ,	
	kənˌtrəʊld 'vɒmɪtɪŋ]	
	bingeing ['bɪndʒɪŋ]	Fressattacke(n)
	hair growth ['heə grəʊθ]	Haarwuchs

enthusiasm [ɪnˈθjuːziæzəm]	Begeisterung	
glossy magazine [ˌglɒsi ˌmægəˈziːn]	Hochglanzmagazin T	
size [saɪz]	Größe T	
overeat [ˌəʊvərˈiːt]	zu viel essen, sich über-fressen T	
soon enough [ˌsuːn ɪˈnʌf]	früh genug T	
spot [spɒt]	erkennen T	
starve sb/sth of sth [ˈstɑːv əv]	jdm/etw etw vorent-halten T	
weight loss [ˈweɪt lɒs]	Gewichtsverlust, -ab-nahme T	
hair loss [ˈheə lɒs]	Haarausfall T	
malnutrition [ˌmælnjuːˈtrɪʃn]	Unterernährung T	
bulimic [buːˈlɪmɪk]	Bulimiker/in T	
horrible [ˈhɒrəbl]	schrecklich, furchtbar T	
family doctor [ˌfæməli ˈdɒktə]	Hausarzt T	

64

63 **sensitive to sth** [ˈsensətɪv tə] auf etw Rücksicht neh-men, einfühlsam sein

encourage [ɪnˈkʌrɪdʒ] fördern

ignore [ɪgˈnɔː] nicht beachten, ignorie-ren

statistics [stəˈtɪstɪks] Statistik(en)

population [ˌpɒpjuˈleɪʃn] Bevölkerung

take steps [ˌteɪk ˈsteps] Schritte unternehmen

address a problem [əˌdres ə ˈprɒbləm] sich mit einem Problem befassen

clinic [ˈklɪnɪk] Klinik

facility [fəˈsɪləti] Einrichtung

generally [ˈdʒenrəli] im Allgemeinen

psychological [ˌsaɪkəˈlɒdʒɪkl] psychologisch

counseling [ˈkaʊnslɪŋ] Beratung

nutritional [njuˈtrɪʃnəl] Ernährungs-

therapy [ˈθerəpi] Therapie

medical attention [ˌmedɪkl əˈtenʃn] ärztliche Behandlung, ärztliche Hilfe

adolescent [ˌædəˈlesnt] heranwachsend, jugend-lich

picky [ˈpɪki] wählerisch

miss sth [mɪs] etw verpassen

chance [tʃɑːns] Gelegenheit, Chance

count [kaʊnt] zählen

weigh [weɪ] abwiegen, wiegen

uncontrolled [ˌʌnkənˈtrəʊld] unkontrolliert

dieting [ˈdaɪətɪŋ] eine Diät machen

extreme [ɪkˈstriːm] extrem

mood swing [ˈmuːd swɪŋ] Stimmungsschwan-kungen

traumatic [trɔːˈmætɪk] traumatisch

abuse [əˈbjuːz] missbrauchen

failure [ˈfeɪljə] Scheitern, Versagen

humiliation [hjuːˌmɪliˈeɪʃn] Demütigung

turn to sth [ˈtɜːn tə] sich einer Sache zuwen-den

in the open [ɪn ðɪ ˈəʊpən] offen

be pushy [bi ˈpʊʃi] zudringlich sein, über-mäßig ehrgeizig sein

foundation [faʊnˈdeɪʃn] Fundament

encourage [ɪnˈkʌrɪdʒ] ermutigen, ermuntern

thought [θɔːt] Gedanke, Überlegung

live up to sth [ˌlɪv ˈʌp tə] einer Sache gerecht werden, etw erfüllen

expectation [ˌekspekˈteɪʃn] Erwartung

primarily [praɪˈmerəli] zu(aller)erst

support [səˈpɔːt] Unterstützung, Hilfe

65 **majority** [məˈdʒɒrəti] Mehrheit, größter Teil

unable [ʌnˈeɪbl] unfähig

unhealthy [ʌnˈhelθi] krankhaft

wonder [ˈwʌndə] sich fragen T

incredible [ɪnˈkredəbl] unglaublich T

hang out with sb [ˌhæŋ ˈaʊt wɪð] sich mit jdm rumtrei-ben T

surely [ˈʃʊəli] sicher(lich), bestimmt T

play a part [ˌpleɪ ə ˈpɑːt] eine Rolle spielen T

soccer (AE) [ˈsɒkə] Fußball T

spending [ˈspendɪŋ] Ausgaben, Etat T

65 **mind** [maɪnd] Verstand, Geist, Kopf

act [ækt] handeln, sich verhalten

self-image [ˌself ˈɪmɪdʒ] Selbstbild

anorexic [ˌænəˈreksɪk] Anorektiker/in

starve oneself [ˈstɑːv wʌnself] hungern

binge [bɪndʒ] sich vollstopfen

guilt [gɪlt] Schuld

meet expectations [ˌmiːt ekspekˈteɪʃnz] Erwartungen erfüllen

power [ˈpaʊə] Kraft, Macht

high [haɪ] *hier:* Hochgefühl

binge [bɪndʒ] Fressattacke

purge [pɜːdʒ] kontrolliertes Vomitie-ren, Erbrechen

fight sb [faɪt] jdn bekämpfen, gegen jdn kämpfen

motivation [ˌməʊtɪˈveɪʃn] Motivation

hopelessness [ˈhəʊpləsnəs] Hoffnungslosigkeit

take your life [ˌteɪk jɔː ˈlaɪf] sich umbringen

66 **underweight** [ˌʌndəˈweɪt] untergewichtig

drug user [ˈdrʌg juːzə] Drogenabhängige/r

officially [əˈfɪʃəli] offiziell

replace [rɪˈpleɪs] ersetzen

unit [ˈjuːnɪt] Einheit

respond [rɪˈspɒnd]	reagieren, *(auf eine Behandlung)* ansprechen	
fried [fraɪd]	gebraten	
fried egg [ˌfraɪd ˈeg]	Spiegelei	
boiled [bɔɪld]	gekocht	
whole milk [ˌhəʊl ˈmɪlk]	Vollmilch	
bacon [ˈbeɪkən]	Speck	
apricot [ˈeɪprɪkɒt]	Aprikose	
date [deɪt]	Dattel	
brazil nut [brəˌzɪl ˈnʌt]	Paranuss	

67	emergency [ɪˈmɜːdʒənsi]	Notfall
	mind [maɪnd]	(etwas) dagegen haben, ausmachen
	alert [əˈlɜːt]	aufgeweckt
	sympathy [ˈsɪmpəθi]	Mitgefühl, Mitleid, Verständnis
	nasty [ˈnɑːsti]	böse, schlimm

68	slim [slɪm]	schlank
	mixed up [ˌmɪkst ˈʌp]	durcheinander, vertauscht
	presenter [prɪˈzentə]	Moderator/in
	fall off [ˌfɔːl ˈɒf]	zurückgehen, nachlassen
	tummy [ˈtʌmi]	Bauch
	flat [flæt]	flach
	excited [ɪkˈsaɪtɪd]	aufgeregt, freudig erregt
	cut back [ˌkʌt ˈbæk]	kürzen, zurückschrauben
	madness [ˈmædnəs]	Irrsinn
	starvation [stɑːˈveɪʃn]	Hungern, Unterernährung
	challenge [ˈtʃælɪndʒ]	Herausforderung, Kampfansage, Wettstreit
	comfort [ˈkʌmfət]	Trost
	obsess about sth [əbˈses əbaʊt]	sich andauernd/zwanghaft mit etw beschäftigen
	permanent [ˈpɜːmənənt]	dauernd
	period [ˈpɪəriəd]	Periode
	risk [rɪsk]	riskieren
	constipation [ˌkɒnstɪˈpeɪʃn]	Verstopfung
	dress size [ˈdres saɪz]	Kleidergröße
	unattractive [ˌʌnəˈtræktɪv]	unattraktiv
	Uruguayan [ˌjʊərəˈgwaɪən]	aus Uruguay
	lettuce leaves [ˈletɪs liːvz]	Salatblätter
	World Health Organization (WHO) [ˌwɜːld ˈhelθ ɔːgənaɪzeɪʃn]	Weltgesundheitsorganisation
	joy (of sth) [dʒɔɪ]	Freude (über etw)
	kick in [ˌkɪk ˈɪn]	einsetzen
	cry [kraɪ]	weinen, heulen
	for no reason	ohne Grund

	[fə ˌnəʊ ˈriːzn]	
	even though [ˈiːvn ðəʊ]	obwohl
	insecure [ˌɪnsɪˈkjʊə]	unsicher, verunsichert
	disaster [dɪˈzɑːstə]	Katastrophe
	jealous [ˈdʒeləs]	eifersüchtig, neidisch
	thinness [ˈθɪnəs]	Schlankheit
	crew [kruː]	Team
	record [rɪˈkɔːd]	aufnehmen, *hier:* filmen
	curvy [ˈkɜːvi]	kurvig
	skinny [ˈskɪni]	mager, dürr
	aim [eɪm]	Ziel, Absicht
	miserable [ˈmɪzrəbl]	elend

69	reality [riˈæləti]	Wirklichkeit
	ban [bæn]	verbieten
	illustrated [ˈɪləstreɪtɪd]	bebildert, illustriert
	guideline [ˈgaɪdlaɪn]	Leitfaden
	spot [spɒt]	entdecken, erkennen

Unit 10

70	reliable [rɪˈlaɪəbl]	zuverlässig
	confident [ˈkɒnfɪdənt]	selbstbewusst
	talkative [ˈtɔːkətɪv]	gesprächig
	cheerful [ˈtʃɪəfl]	gut gelaunt, fröhlich
	well-organized [ˌwel ˈɔːgənaɪzd]	gut organisiert
	responsible [rɪˈspɒnsəbl]	verantwortungsbewusst
	dislike [dɪsˈlaɪk]	nicht mögen
	hate [heɪt]	hassen, überhaupt nicht mögen
	stand [stænd]	ertragen
	work overtime [ˌwɜːk ˈəʊvətaɪm]	Überstunden machen
	hectic [ˈhektɪk]	Hektik
	rude [ruːd]	unhöflich, unverschämt

71	vocational qualification [vəʊˌkeɪʃnəl kwɒlɪfɪˈkeɪʃn]	Berufsabschluss
	assess [əˈses]	festsetzen, einschätzen
	gain [geɪn]	*(Kenntnisse)* erwerben
	night school [ˈnaɪt skuːl]	Abendschule
	self-study [ˌself ˈstʌdi]	Selbststudium
	registered [ˈredʒɪstəd]	registriert
	approved [əˈpruːvd]	anerkannt
	council [ˈkaʊnsl]	Rat
	midwifery [ˌmɪdˈwaɪfəri]	Geburtshilfe
	foundation [faʊnˈdeɪʃn]	Basis
	degree [dɪˈgriː]	Abschluss
	membership [ˈmembəʃɪp]	Mitgliedschaft
	membership organization [ˈmembəʃɪp ɔːgənaɪzeɪʃn]	Fachverband, Berufsverband
	column [ˈkɒləm]	Spalte
	responsible for [rɪˈspɒnsəbl]	verantwortlich, zuständig für
	organize [ˈɔːgənaɪz]	organisieren

work routine ['wɜːk ruːtiːn]	Arbeitsablauf	
require [rɪ'kwaɪə]	erfordern, verlangen, voraussetzen	
apply to sb for sth [ə'plaɪ]	sich bei jdm um etw bewerben	
experienced [ɪk'spɪəriənst]	erfahren	
assessment [ə'sesmənt]	Einschätzung, Beurteilung	
assessment skills [ə'sesmənt skɪlz]	Einschätzungsvermögen	
decision-making [dɪ'sɪʒn meɪkɪŋ]	Entscheidungsfindung	
range [reɪndʒ]	Reihe, Auswahl	
desirable [dɪ'zaɪərəbl]	erwünscht	
evidence ['evɪdəns]	Nachweis	
professional [prə'feʃnəl]	beruflich	
target ['tɑːgɪt]	Ziel, Zielvorgabe	
specified ['spesɪfaɪd]	festgelegt	
standard ['stændəd]	Anforderung, Richtlinie, Norm	
care assistant [ˌkeər ə'sɪstənt]	Pflegeassistent/in	
interpersonal skills [ˌɪntə'pɜːsnəl skɪlz]	soziale Kompetenz	
applicant ['æplɪkənt]	Bewerber/in	
smart [smɑːt]	intelligent, aufgeweckt	
enthusiastic about sth [ɪn,θjuːzi'æstɪk əbaʊt]	von etw begeistert	
in writing [ɪn 'raɪtɪŋ]	schriftlich	
nursing home ['nɜːsɪŋ həʊm]	Pflegeheim	
require [rɪ'kwaɪə]	benötigen	
handle ['hændl]	erledigen	
inquiry [ɪn'kwaɪəri]	Anfrage	
manage ['mænɪdʒ]	verwalten	

72 **previous** ['priːviəs]	vorhergehend, vorig	
... and stuff [ənd ˌstʌf]	und so T	
make use of [ˌmeɪk 'juːs əv]	nutzen T	
leader ['liːdə]	Leiter/in T	
post-graduate diploma [pəʊstˌgrædʒuət dɪ'pləʊmə]	weiterführender Studienabschluss T	
be about to do sth [bi ə'baʊt tə duː]	dabei sein, etw zu tun T	
as well [əz 'wel]	auch T	
temping agency ['tempɪŋ eɪdʒənsi]	Zeitarbeitsfirma T	
temporary ['temprəri]	vorübergehend, (Arbeit:) befristet T	
secretarial [ˌsekrə'teəriəl]	Sekretariats- T	
get on with sb [ˌget 'ɒn wɪð]	mit jdm zurechtkommen T	
pretty ['prɪti]	ziemlich T	
application [ˌæplɪ'keɪʃn]	Bewerbung	

letter of application [ˌletər əv æplɪ'keɪʃn]	Bewerbungsschreiben	
advertise ['ædvətaɪz]	annoncieren, (Stelle) ausschreiben	
department store [dɪ'pɑːtmənt stɔː]	Kaufhaus	
sales target ['seɪlz tɑːgɪt]	Umsatzziel, Verkaufsziel	
enclosed [ɪn'kləʊzd]	(Brief:) beigefügt	
curriculum vitae (CV) [kə,rɪkjələm 'viːtaɪ]	Lebenslauf	
doctor's assistant [ˌdɒktəz ə'sɪstənt]	medizinische/r Fachangestellte/r	
marry ['mæri]	heiraten	
interest ['ɪntrəst]	interessieren	
advertisement [əd'vɜːtɪsmənt]	Anzeige, Annonce	
be available for sth [bi ə'veɪləbl fə]	für etw zur Verfügung stehen	
look forward to sth [ˌlʊk 'fɔːwəd tə]	sich auf etw freuen	
Yours sincerely [jɔːz sɪn'sɪəli]	(Brief:) Mit freundlichen Grüßen	
enc(losures) [ɪn'kləʊʒəz]	(Brief:) Anlagen	

73 **education** [ˌedʒu'keɪʃn]	Schulbildung	
rest (with sth) ['rest wɪð]	(auf etw) ruhen	
career ladder [kə'rɪə lædə]	Karriereleiter	
therefore ['ðeəfɔː]	daher	
represent [ˌreprɪ'zent]	darstellen, repräsentieren	
miss out on sth [ˌmɪs 'aʊt ɒn]	sich etw entgehen lassen	
reader ['riːdə]	Leser/in	
attract sb's attention [ə,trækt ˌsʌmbədiz ə'tenʃn]	jds Aufmerksamkeit wecken	
employer [ɪm'plɔɪə]	Arbeitgeber/in	
invite [ɪn'vaɪt]	einladen	
move on to sth [muːv 'ɒn tə]	zu etw übergehen	
appropriate [ə'prəʊpriət]	angemessen, passend	
section break ['sekʃn breɪk]	Abschnittswechsel	
hand-written [ˌhænd 'rɪtn]	handgeschrieben	
typewriter ['taɪpraɪtə]	Schreibmaschine	
old fashioned [ˌəʊld 'fæʃənd]	altmodisch	
out of date [ˌaʊt əv 'deɪt]	veraltet, überholt	
requirement [rɪ'kwaɪəmənt]	Anforderung, Bedürfnis	
interview sb ['ɪntəvjuː]	mit jdm ein Vorstellungsgespräch führen	
date of birth [ˌdeɪt əv 'bɜːθ]	Geburtsdatum	
marital status [ˌmærɪtl 'steɪtəs]	Familienstand	
nationality [ˌnæʃə'næləti]	Staatsangehörigkeit	

abroad [ə'brɔːd] — im Ausland

professional association [prə,feʃnəl əsəʊsi'eɪʃn] — Berufsverband

subject ['sʌbdʒɪkt] — (Schul-, Studien-)Fach

relevant to ['reləvənt tə] — relevant für, wichtig für

backwards ['bækwədz] — rückwärts

responsibility [rɪ,spɒnsə'bɪləti] — Verantwortlichkeit, Zuständigkeit

achievement [ə'tʃiːvmənt] — Leistung, Errungenschaft, Erfolg

transfer [træns'fɜː] — übertragen

foreign language skills [,fɒrən 'læŋgwɪdʒ skɪlz] — Fremdsprachenkenntnisse

indicate ['ɪndɪkeɪt] — angeben

technical ['teknɪkl] — technisch, Fach-

strength [streŋθ] — Stärke

specific [spə'sɪfɪk] — konkret, genau

versatile ['vɜːsətaɪl] — vielseitig

motivate ['məʊtɪveɪt] — motivieren

staff appraisal [,stɑːf ə'preɪzl] — Mitarbeiterbeurteilung

reference ['refərəns] — Referenz, Zeugnis

surprising [sə'praɪzɪŋ] — überraschend

74 additional [ə'dɪʃnəl] — zusätzlich, Zusatz-

present ['preznt] — Gegenwart

sales area [,seɪlz 'eəriə] — Verkaufsfläche

stock levels ['stɒk levlz] — Lagerbestände

sandwich release (course) [,sænwɪdʒ rɪ'liːs kɔːs] — Kurs mit abwechselnder theoretischer und praktischer Ausbildung

native speaker [,neɪtɪv 'spiːkə] — Muttersprachler/in

be fluent in sth [bi 'fluːənt ɪn] — etw fließend sprechen können

intermediate French [ɪntə,miːdiət 'frentʃ] — Französisch auf fortgeschrittenem Anfängerniveau

driving licence ['draɪvɪŋ laɪsns] — Führerschein

75 attach [ə'tætʃ] — (Brief:) beifügen

present ['preznt] — gegenwärtig, aktuell

reply [rɪ'plaɪ] — Antwort

76 career advisor [kə'rɪər ədvaɪzə] — Berufsberater/in, Karriereberater/in

recommendation [,rekəmen'deɪʃn] — Empfehlung

in advance [ɪn əd'vɑːns] — im voraus

relaxing bath [rɪ,læksɪŋ 'bɑːθ] — Entspannungsbad

stay awake [,steɪ ə'weɪk] — wach bleiben

stressful ['stresfl] — anstrengend, stressig T

preparation [,prepə'reɪʃn] — Vorbereitung T

beforehand [bɪ'fɔːhænd] — vorher T

traffic ['træfɪk] — (Straßen-)Verkehr T

sensible ['sensəbl] — vernünftig T

Practice makes perfect. [,præktɪs meɪks 'pɜːfɪkt] — Übung macht den Meister. T

appearance [ə'pɪərəns] — (äußere) Erscheinung, Erscheinungsbild T

smart [smɑːt] — (Kleidung:) schick T

skydiving ['skaɪdaɪvɪŋ] — Fallschirmspringen

employee [ɪm'plɔɪiː] — Angestellte/r

interviewer [,ɪntəvjuːə] — Interviewer/in

interviewee [,ɪntəvjuː'iː] — Befragte/r, Bewerber(in)

trainer ['treɪnə] — Ausbilder/in

role-play ['rəʊl pleɪ] — Rollenspiel

77 retail ['riːteɪl] — Einzelhandel

nerve-racking ['nɜːv rækɪŋ] — nervenaufreibend

have your say in sth [həv jɔː 'seɪ ɪn] — seine Meinung zu etw äußern

pay [peɪ] — Gehalt, Lohn, Bezahlung

A–Z Word list

Diese Liste enthält alle Wörter in alphabetischer Reihenfolge. Es sind jedoch die Wörter, die zum Grundwortschtz gehören, hier nicht aufgeführt. (Siehe Basic word list.)
T = das Wort befindet sich im Transkripte der Hörverständnistexte.

A

ability *13*   Fähigkeit
able: be ~ to *57*   in der Lage sein
about: be ~ to do sth *72T* dabei sein, etw zu tun
abroad *73*   im Ausland
absolutely *46T*   völlig, absolut, ganz
abuse *63*   missbrauchen
accept *33*   akzeptieren
according to *48*   laut, nach, gemäß
accurate *13*   genau, akkurat
ache *22*   schmerzen
achieve *11*   erreichen, erlangen
achievement *73*   Leistung, Errungenschaft, Erfolg
acronym *20*   Abkürzung, Akronym
across *31*   auf der anderen Seite von/des; **across Europe** *25*   in ganz Europa
act *60*   spielen; *65*   handeln, sich verhalten
active *38*   aktiv; **keep sb ~** *61*   jdn auf Trab halten
activity *12*   Tätigkeit
actual *28*   wirklich, tatsächlich
actually *47T*   wirklich, tatsächlich
add *13*   hinzufügen
additional *74*   zusätzlich, Zusatz-
address a problem *63*   sich mit einem Problem befassen
adequate *38*   angemessen
administrative staff *13*   Verwaltungspersonal
adolescent *63*   heranwachsend, jugendlich
advance: in ~ *76*   im voraus
advertise *72*   annoncieren, *(Stelle)* ausschreiben
advertisement *72*   Anzeige, Annonce

advice *44*   (guter) Rat, Ratschlag; **~ column** *62*   *(Zeitschrift:)* Kummerkasten
advise *51*   raten, beraten
affect *11*   beeinflussen; *55*   betreffen; *57*   beeinträchtigen
afraid: be ~ of sth *42*   vor etw Angst haben
aged *38*   im Alter von
agency *38*   Agentur, Behörde
agree *23*   zustimmen
aim *68*   Ziel, Absicht
air *21T*   Luft
alert *67*   aufgeweckt
allergic *17*   allergisch
allow *61*   gestatten, erlauben; **~ to dissolve** *34*   zergehen lassen; **be ~ed to do sth** *13*   etw tun dürfen
almost *18*   fast, beinah
alter *61*   verändern
although *61*   obwohl
ambulance *25*   Rettungswagen
among *38*   unter
amongst *25*   unter, bei
amount *35T*   Menge
amplify *21*   verstärken
anaesthetic *17T*   Betäubungsmittel
analysis, analyses *54T*   Analyse, Analysen
angry *47T*   ungehalten, wütend
ankle *30*   (Fuß-)Knöchel
anorexia *62*   Anorexie
anorexic *65*   Anorektiker/in
antibiotics *19*   Antibiotika
anti-depressant *32*   Antidepressivum
antiseptic *35*   antiseptisch
anvil *21*   Amboss
anxiety *41*   Angst, Sorge
anxious *17*   besorgt, ängstlich, nervös
anything in particular *49T* etwas Besonderes
anyway *21T*   also, wie dem auch sei
apologize *47T*   sich entschuldigen
appear *60*   auftreten
appearance *76T*   (äußere) Erscheinung, Erscheinungsbild
appendix *30*   Blinddarm
appliance *13*   Gerät
applicant *71*   Bewerber/in

application *72*   Bewerbung; **letter of ~** *72*   Bewerbungsschreiben
apply to sb for sth *20*   sich bei jdm um etw bewerben
appointment *6*   Termin; **~ book** *20*   Terminkalender; **~ card** *15*   Terminzettel
appropriate *73*   angemessen, passend
approved *71*   anerkannt
apricot *66*   Aprikose
arise *61*   auftreten, auftauchen
arrange *37*   arrangieren, vereinbaren
arrive *35T*   ankommen, eintreffen
artery *43*   Arterie; **~ forceps** *43*   Arterienklemme
article *25*   Artikel
as: as if *31*   als ob; **as long as** *35T*   solange; **as well** *72T*   auch
assess *71*   festsetzen, einschätzen
assessment *71*   Einschätzung, Beurteilung; **~ skills** *71*   Einschätzungsvermögen
assignment *11*   Aufgabe; **work-based ~** *11*   praktische Prüfungsaufgabe
assist sb *12*   jdm assistieren
(shop) assistant *33*   Verkäufer/in
associate sb with sth *42*   jdn mit etw in Verbindung bringen
assume the worst *54*   das Schlimmste befürchten
at all *20*   überhaupt
atmosphere *42*   Atmosphäre, Stimmung
attach *15*   befestigen; *75* *(Brief:)* beifügen
attack *59T*   Anfall, Attacke; *56* angreifen, befallen
attract sb's attention *73*   jds Aufmerksamkeit wecken
auditory nerve *21*   Hörnerv
Australian *^9*   Australier/in
author *61*   Autor/in, Verfasser/in
available *11*   verfügbar, erhältlich; **be ~ for sth** *72*   für etw zur Verfügung stehen

average *11* Durchschnitt, Durchschnitts-
avoid *47* vermeiden
awake: stay ~ *76* wach bleiben
award-winning *53* preisgekrönt
awareness *25* Bewusstsein
awful *40T* schrecklich, fürchterlich

B
back *21T* Rückseite, hinterer Teil; *30* Rücken
backache *24* Rückenschmerzen
background *13* Herkunft, Hintergrund
backwards *73* rückwärts
bacon *66* Speck
balance *21* Gleichgewicht
ban *69* verbieten
bandage *24T* Verband
bang *56* knallen
bargain *37* Schnäppchen
beach *40T* Strand
because of *53* wegen
beef *49T* Rind(fleisch)
beforehand *76T* vorher
behave: be badly ~d *48* sich schlecht benehmen, unartig sein
belief *38* Glaube, Überzeugung
believe *25* glauben
below *9* unten(stehend); *50* unterhalb
bend *55* beugen
benefit *44T* Nutzen, Vorteil
bike *18* Fahrrad
binge *65* Fressattacke; *65* sich vollstopfen
bingeing *62* Fressattacke(n)
biscuit *49* Keks
black market *53* Schwarzmarkt
bladder *54T* Blase
blanket *56* Decke
blister *24* Blase
blocked *23T* verstopft
blood *8* Blut
blood glucose control *51* Blutzuckerregulation
blood glucose level *51* Blutzuckerspiegel
blood pressure *26* Blutdruck; ~ cuff *26* Blutdruckmanschette; take ~ *29* den Blutdruck messen

blood sample *28* Blutprobe
blood test *8* Blutuntersuchung
blurred vision *34* verschwommenes Sehen
body *21T* Körper
boiled *66* gekocht
bone *21* Knochen
book *11* buchen
booth *31* Kabine
both ... and *11* sowohl ... als auch
bottle *35* Flasche
bowel *54T* Darm
bra *56* BH
bracket *55* Klammer
brain *20* Gehirn, Hirn
brazil nut *66* Paranuss
bread roll *49* Brötchen
break *18* brechen; Bruch
breast *46T* Brust
breath *25* Atem; short of ~ *55* außer Atem
breathe *22* atmen
broad *39* breit
broadband *31* Breitband
broken *26* ge-, zerbrochen
bronchoscope *43* Bronchoskop
bruise *24* blauer Fleck, Prellung
brush *46T* Bürste, Pinsel
bubble *53* (Luft-)Blase
building *13* Gebäude
bulimia *62* Bulimie
bulimic *62T* Bulimiker/in
burn a candle *44T* eine Kerze verwenden, brennen lassen
bus station *36* Busbahnhof
businessman *41* Geschäftsmann
busy: be ~ *6* viel zu tun haben
buttocks *30* Gesäß, Hinterbacken

C
cabbage *49T* Kohl
calendar *15* Kalender
call *25* rufen; call up *35T* aufrufen
called *20* namens
caller *7* Anrufer/in
calm *25* ruhig
calorie *48* Kalorie
campaign *53* Kampagne, Aktion
cancer *42* Krebs
candle *44* Kerze
candy *37* Süßigkeiten

capsule *33* Kapsel
car crash *55* Autounfall
car park *36* Parkplatz
carbohydrates *48* Kohlenhydrate
carbonated *53* kohlensäurehaltig
card reader port *15* Kartenlesegerät
cardiologist *23* Kardiologe/-in
care *47* Betreuung, Pflege; ~ assistant *71* Pflegeassistent/in; take ~ of sb *47T* auf jdn aufpassen, sich um jdn kümmern
career *61* Beruf, Laufbahn, Karriere; ~ advisor *76* Berufsberater/in, Karriereberater/in; ~ ladder *73* Karriereleiter
careful: be ~ of sth *20* auf etw achten, auf etw aufpassen
carefully *43* sorgfältig, genau
carer *47* Betreuer/in, Pfleger/in
caring *11* sozial (eingestellt)
carry *21T* befördern
carry on *61* weitermachen
carry out *25* durchführen
cart *37* Karren
cartilage *21* Knorpel
case *34* Fall; ~ study *61* Fallstudie
cash box *15* Kasse
catch one's breath *25* Luft/Atem holen
catch sth *42* sich mit etw anstecken
cause *22* verursachen
cause *42* Ursache, Grund
cell *46T* Zelle; ~ death *57* Zelltod
central *57* zentral
cereal *49* Getreide, Getreideflocken
certainly *7T* sicherlich
cervix *46T* Gebärmutterhals
chain *21* Kette
challenge *68* Herausforderung, Kampfansage, Wettstreit
challenging *11* fordernd, anspruchsvoll
chance *63* Gelegenheit, Chance
change *52T* Änderung, Veränderung; *51* (sich) verändern, (sich) ändern
channel sth *21* etw leiten

charge _20_ Ladung

charity _38_ Wohlfahrtsorganisation

chart _49_ Grafik

cheap _37_ billig, preiswert

check _16T_ überprüfen

check-up _12_ (Vorsorge-)
Untersuchung

cheerful _70_ gut gelaunt,
fröhlich

chef _53_ Koch/Köchin

chest _19_ Brust

chest infection _52T_ Lungeninfekt

chesty cough _32T_ bronchialer
Husten

chicken _49_ Huhn

chin _30_ Kinn

Chinese _40_ chinesisch

chips _53_ Pommes frites

cholesterol _50_ Cholesterin;
~ **level** _50_ Cholesterinspiegel

choose _8_ wählen

circulation _62_ Kreislauf,
Zirkulation

clasp _56_ Verschluss, Schließe

client _47_ Klient/in, Kunde/
Kundin

clinic _63_ Klinik

clinical _13_ klinisch

close _13_ schließen, abschlie-
ßen; _31_ nahe, dicht

close by _18_ nahe gelegen

coach _51_ Reisebus

cochlea _21_ Hörschnecke

coconut _49_ Kokosnuss

cold _32T_ Erkältung

cold cut _49_ Aufschnitt

coldness _42_ Kälte

collect _13_ sammeln, kassieren

column _71_ Spalte

come down with _32T_ _(eine_
Krankheit) bekommen,
kriegen

comfort _68_ Trost

comfortable _20_ angenehm;
Are you ~? _56_ _hier:_ Liegen
Sie bequem?

common _42_ üblich, verbreitet

commonly _51_ häufig, gewöhnlich

community _13_ Gemeinde

company _16T_ Gesellschaft,
Firma

compare _35_ vergleichen

compared with _25_ verglichen
mit

complete _9_ ausfüllen; _10_

vervollständigen; _23_ ab-
schließen; _14_ vollständig

condition _50_ Zustand

conduct _31_ durchführen

confectionery foods _51_ Süßwaren, Konditoreierzeugnisse

confident _70_ selbstbewusst

connect _21_ verbinden

conscious _25_ bewusst

considerable _25_ erheblich

constant _61_ ständig

constipation _68_ Verstopfung

consult _24_ konsultieren; beraten

consultant _23_ Facharzt/-ärztin

consume _49_ verzehren

contagious _51_ ansteckend

contain _48_ enthalten

content _38_ Inhalt

continually _38_ stetig, kontinu-
ierlich

continue to do sth _61_ etw
weiterhin tun

contraceptive _32_ empfängnisverhütend, Empfängnisverhü-
tungsmittel

contrast: in ~ _57_ im Gegensatz
dazu, dagegen

contribute _25_ beitragen

control _42_ Kontrolle; _21_
kontrollieren; _52_ regulieren

copy _10_ abschreiben

corner _36_ Ecke

coronary heart disease _25_
koronare Herzerkrankung

corridor _16T_ Flur

cosmetics _32_ Kosmetika

cotton _26_ Baumwolle

cotton swab _26_ Wattetupfer

cottonwool _28T_ Watte

cough _23T_ Husten; husten;
~ **mixture** _32_ Hustensaft;
~ **sweet** _32_ Hustenbonbon

council _71_ Rat

counseling _63_ Beratung

count _63_ zählen

counter: over-the-~ _32_ frei
verkäuflich

couple: a ~ of _27_ ein paar

course _11_ Kurs; _59T_ Verlauf;
of ~ _21T_ natürlich

cover _33_ _(Kosten)_ decken

crazy _52T_ verrückt

cream _49_ Sahne

create _31_ schaffen

crew _68_ Team

crisis, crises _39_ Krise, Krisen

cross _36T_ überqueren

crossroads _36T_ Kreuzung

crutches _18_ Krücken

cry _68_ weinen, heulen

culture _6_ Kultur

cure _38_ Heilmittel; Heilung,
Therapie; _38_ heilen

currently _57_ derzeit, zurzeit,
momentan

curriculum vitae (CV) _72_ Le-
benslauf

curvy _68_ kurvig

customer _33_ Kunde/Kundin

cut _18_ Schnitt, Schnittverletzung

cut back _68_ kürzen, zurück-
schrauben

cut your arm _18_ sich in den
Arm schneiden

cutaway _55_ Schnittbild,
Schnittansicht

D

dairy products _49_ Molkerei-
produkte, Milchprodukte

damage _52T_ Schaden, Schäden

danger _52_ Gefahr

dangerous _50_ gefährlich

database _47_ Datenbank

date _15_ Datum; _66_ Dattel;
~ **of birth** _73_ Geburtsdatum;
~ **stamp** _15_ Datumsstempel;
out of ~ _73_ veraltet, überholt

day-to-day _52T_ täglich

deaf _18_ taub

deal with sb _9_ mit jdm umgehen, sich um jdn kümmern

deal with sth _25_ zu tun haben
mit; _54_ mit etw umgehen,
mit etw fertig werden, mit etw
zurecht kommen

death _41_ Tod

decide _48_ entscheiden

decision-making _71_ Entschei-
dungsfindung

decline _59T_ Rückgang

deep _24T_ tief

definite _59T_ sicher, bestimmt,
definitiv

degree _71_ Abschluss

delicious _37_ delikat, lecker

deliver _35T_ liefern

delivery _16T_ Lieferung;
~ **note** _16T_ Lieferschein

dental _41_ Zahn-

department store _72_ Kaufhaus

depressed _54T_ niedergeschla-
gen, deprimiert

describe *14* beschreiben
description *13* Beschreibung
design *25* gestalten, entwerfen
desirable *71* erwünscht
despite *53* trotz
destroy *53* zerstören
detail: in ~ *46T* im einzelnen
details *9* Angaben, Einzelheiten
develop *51* entwickeln
development *57* Entwicklung
device *31* Gerät
diabetes *51* Diabetes
diagnose *12* diagnostizieren
diagnosis, diagnoses *38*
  Diagnose, Diagnosen; **make
  a ~** *22* eine Diagnose stellen
diagram *21* Grafik
diarrhoea *23T* Durchfall
dictionary *17* Wörterbuch
die *25* sterben
diet *48* Ernährung, Kost
dieting *63* eine Diät machen
difference *11* Unterschied; *18*
  verschieden, unterschiedlich
difficult *31* schwierig
dignity *13* Würde
diner *37* Imbissstube, Lokal
diploma *11* Diplom
direction *27T* Richtung; **give
  ~s** *16* den Weg beschreiben
director *25* Direktor/in
disability *47* Behinderung
disabled *40* behindert
disagree *23* nicht zustimmen
disaster *68* Katastrophe
discomfort *43* Unbehagen,
  Schmerz
discover *25* entdecken, herausfinden
discuss *23* diskutieren,
  erörtern
disease *23* Krankheit
disinfect *24T* desinfizieren
disinfectant *26* Desinfektions-
  mittel
dislike *70* nicht mögen
disorder *62* Störung
disposable *35* Einweg-
dissolve *34* auflösen; **allow
  to ~** *34* zergehen lassen
divided by *62* geteilt durch
dizzy *25* schwindlig
do exercise *51* sich bewegen,
  Sport treiben
doctor's assistant *72* medizi-
  nische/r Fachangestellte/r
dormant *60* ruhend, nicht
  aktiv

dosage *32T* Dosierung
dose *35* Dosis
dramatically *57* drastisch
dress a wound *26* eine Wunde
  verbinden
dress size *68* Kleidergröße
dressing *24* Verband
driving licence *74* Führerschein
drop *33* Tropfen; *53* Rückgang
drowsiness *34* Schläfrigkeit
drug *17* Arzneimittel, Medikament
drug user *66* Drogenabhän-
  gige/r
dry *32T* trocken
due: be ~ to sth *38* auf etw
  zurückzuführen sein
during *44* während
duties *13* Aufgaben

E
ear Ohr; ~ **canal** *21* Gehörgang; ~ **wax** *18* Ohrenschmalz
earache *24* Ohrenschmerzen
eardrum *21* Trommelfell
earplug *56* Ohrstöpsel
ease *57* lindern
eating disorder *62* Essstörung
education *73* Schulbildung
educational *13* Ausbildungs-
effect: take ~ *27* wirken, Wirkung zeigen
effervescent tablet *33* Brausetablette
efficient *13* effizient
either ... or *11* entweder ...
  oder
elastic bandage *26* elastische
  Binde
elbow *30* Ellbogen
(the) elderly *47* ältere Men-
  schen, Senioren
electrical *20* elektrisch
electrocardiograph (ECG) *20*
  Elektrokardiogramm (EKG)
electroencephalograph (EEG)
  20 Elektroenzephalogramm
  (EEG)
electromyogram (EMG) *20*
  Elektromyogramm (EMG)
emergency *67* Notfall
emigrant *41* Auswanderer
emotion *43* Gefühl, Emotion
employee *76* Angestellte/r
employer *73* Arbeitgeber/in

empty *34* leer
enc(losures) *72* *(Brief:)*
  Anlagen
enclosed *72* *(Brief:)* beigefügt
encourage *63* ermutigen,
  ermuntern; *63* fördern
enjoy *11* genießen, gern tun
enthusiasm *62* Begeisterung
enthusiastic about sth *71* von
  etw begeistert
environment *11* Umfeld,
  Umgebung
environmental *51* Umwelt-
equally *51* gleich, gleichermaßen
equipment *15* Ausstattung,
  Geräte
especially *38* besonders
essential *47T* wesentlich, notwendig
Eustachian tube *21* Eustachi-
  Röhre
even though *68* obwohl
evidence *71* Nachweis
exactly *24T* genau
examination/exam *11* Prüfung
examination couch *39* Behandlungsliege
examine *24* untersuchen
excellent *13* ausgezeichnet
excited *68* aufgeregt, freudig
  erregt
exercise *36T* Bewegung,
  Sport; *18* trainieren; **do ~** *51*
  sich bewegen, Sport treiben
expect *44T* erwarten
expectation *63* Erwartung
expensive *56* teuer
experience *13* Erfahrung; *31*
  Erlebnis; *38* erleben, erfahren
experienced *71* erfahren
experiment *31* Versuch,
  Experiment
expert *48* Experte/-in,
  Fachmann/-frau
explain *21* erklären, erläutern
explanation *40* Erklärung,
  Erläuterung
express *35T* per Eilbote
express *41* ausdrücken
external *21* äußere/r/s
extract *26* herausziehen
extreme *25* Extrem; *63*
  extrem

F

face-to-face *31* direkt, persönlich

face: be ~d with sb *43* mit jdm konfrontiert werden

facility *63* Einrichtung

fact *42* Tatsache

fail to do sth *38* versäumen, etw zu tun

failure *63* Scheitern, Versagen

Fair enough. *35T* Na gut. Einverstanden.

fall off *68* zurückgehen, nachlassen

false *6* falsch

family doctor *62T* Hausarzt

fancy sth *37* Lust auf etw haben

far from over *53* noch lange nicht vorbei

fat *49* Fett

fax machine *15* Fax(gerät)

fear *41* Furcht, Angst

fee *13* Honorar, Gebühr

feed *53* ernähren, verpflegen

feel uncomfortable *41* sich unwohl fühlen

feeling *11* Gefühl

fever *23T* Fieber

fibre *50* Ballaststoffe; **high in ~** *50* ballaststoffreich

fight *53* Kampf; *53* kämpfen; **~ sb** *65* jdn bekämpfen, gegen jdn kämpfen; **~ back** *61* sich wehren

file *15* *(Akten)* ablegen

filing cabinet *15* Aktenschrank

fill a prescription *32* ein Rezept dispensieren

fill in *56* *(Formular)* ausfüllen

filled *21* gefüllt

final line *61* letzte Zeile

finally *17T* zuletzt, als letztes

finally *27* schließlich, zum Schluss

find *38* herausfinden, feststellen; *57* entdecken, herausfinden; **~ out** *22* herausfinden

fine: I'm ~. *8* Mir geht es gut.

finished *21T* fertig

finishing point *36* Ziel

fit *61* fit, in Form

fit *52* passen; **fit sb in** *6* jdn dazwischenschieben

fix *15* befestigen

flat *68* flach

flight of stairs *25* Treppe

flu / influenza *23* Grippe

flu jab *51* Grippeimpfung

fluent: be ~ in sth *74* etw fließend sprechen können

fluid *21* Flüssigkeit

focus on sth *57* sich auf etw konzentrieren

foetus *49T* Fötus

folic acid *49T* Folsäure

following *13* folgende/r/s

food poisoning *23* Lebensmittelvergiftung

foot: on ~ *36T* zu Fuß; **~ spa** *44* Fußbad

for no reason *68* ohne Grund

foreign *17* ausländisch

foreign language skills *73* Fremdsprachenkenntnisse

forget *38* vergessen

form *9* Formular

foundation *25* Stiftung; *63* Fundament; *71* Basis

frequent *59T* häufig

fried *66* gebraten; **~ egg** *66* Spiegelei

friendly *42* freundlich

front *21T* Vorderseite, vorderer Teil

frustrated *47T* frustriert

full fat milk *50* Vollmilch

full time *11* Vollzeit-

function *21* Funktion

future *31* Zukunft; *59T* zukünftig

G

gain *71* *(Kenntnisse)* erwerben; **~ a pass** *11* eine Prüfung bestehen

galanin *57* Galanin

gauze dressing *26* Mull-, Gazeverband

gay *38* schwul

general *12* allgemein

general practice *11* Allgemeinarztpraxis

General Practitioner (GP) *9* Allgemeinarzt/-ärztin

generally *63* im Allgemeinen

genetic *51* genetisch, erblich

gentle *39* sanft

germ *40T* Keim, Bakterie

get: ~ on with sth *61* mit etw vorankommen; **~ on with sb** *72T* mit jdm zurechtkommen; **~ some rest** *22* sich ausruhen; **~ started** *56* anfangen

give directions *16* den Weg beschreiben

glad *28T* froh

gland *22* Drüse

glossy magazine *62T* Hochglanzmagazin

gloves *26* Handschuhe

go by *61* vorübergehen, vergehen

gold medal *51* Goldmedaille

gone *38* weg, verschwunden

goodness: My ~. *35T* Meine Güte!

government *53* Regierung

gown *56* Kittel

gradient coils *55* Neigungsspulen

grain *50* Korn

greet *13* begrüßen

grow *38* wachsen, zunehmen, steigen

grow worse *59T* sich verschlimmern

guess *24* raten, erraten

guideline *69* Leitfaden; **guidelines** *53* Richtlinien

guilt *65* Schuld

gullet *21* Speiseröhre

gynaecologist *12* Gynäkologe/-in

H

habit *53* Gewohnheit

hair: ~ growth *62* Haarwuchs; **~ loss** *62T* Haarausfall

hand over *60* übergeben

handle *71* erledigen

hands-on *31* praktisch, direkt

hand-written *73* handgeschrieben

hang out with sb *64T* sich mit jdm rumtreiben

happen *24T* passieren, geschehen

hardly *27T* kaum

harm *49T* schädigen, schaden

harmful *49* schädlich

hate *70* hassen, überhaupt nicht mögen

head *18* Kopf; *38* Chef/in

head office *35* Zentrale, Hauptsitz

headache *23T* Kopfschmerzen

heading *21* Überschrift

heal *24T* heilen, verheilen

health *6* Gesundheit

health and social care *47* Gesundheitswesen und Sozialfürsorge

health care *9* Gesundheitswesen; *9* medizinische Versorgung

health centre *7T* Gesundheitszentrum

health insurance *6* Krankenversicherung

health protection *38* Gesundheitsschutz, -vorsorge

healthy *48* gesund

hearing aid *40* Hörgerät

heart *20* Herz; ~ **attack** *25* Herzinfarkt; ~ **beat** *26* Herzschlag; ~ **disease** *25* Herzerkrankung; ~ **rate** *25* Puls, Herzfrequenz

hectic *70* Hektik

height *62* Körpergröße

helpful *13* hilfsbereit

helpless *42* hilflos

helplessness *43* Hilflosigkeit

hepatitis *17* Hepatitis

high *22* erhöht; *65* Hochgefühl

high-definition *31* hochauflösend

high-fibre *49* ballaststoffreich

highlight *21* hervorheben

hip *30* Hüfte

Hold on. *35T* Einen Moment.

hold out *24T* hinhalten

honest *47* ehrlich, aufrichtig

honesty *47T* Ehrlichkeit, Aufrichtigkeit

honey *50* Honig

hopelessness *65* Hoffnungslosigkeit

horizon *57* Horizont

horrible *62T* schrecklich, furchtbar

human *47T* menschlich

humiliation *63* Demütigung

hurry up *55* sich beeilen

hurt *20* wehtun

hypodermic (syringe) *26* (Injektions-)Spritze

I

ID (card) *16T* Personalausweis

identify *26* identifizieren, erkennen, benennen

ignorance *38* Unkenntnis, Unwissen

ignore *63* nicht beachten, ignorieren

ill *42* krank

illness *18* Krankheit

ill-tempered *47T* griesgrämig, verärgert

illustrated *69* bebildert, illustriert

illustration *15* Abbildung

image *31* Bild

imaging *55* Bildgebung

immediately *6* sofort

immune system *57* Immunsystem

immunization *28* Impfung, Immunisierung

importance *13* Bedeutung, Wichtigkeit

important *11* wichtig, bedeutend

impression *11* Eindruck

improve *50* (sich) bessern, verbessern

improvement *44* Verbesserung

include *13* einschließen, beinhalten

inconvenience sb *6* jdm Umstände bereiten

increase *25* zunehmen; *38* Steigerung

increase *57* ansteigen

incredible *64T* unglaublich

indicate *73* angeben

infection *19* Infektion

inflamed *22* entzündet

infusion *35* Infusion

inject *26* injizieren

injection *14* Injektion, Spritze

injure *57* verletzen

ink *15* einfärben

inkpad *15* Stempelkissen

inner ear *21* Innenohr

inquiry *71* Anfrage

insecure *68* unsicher, verunsichert

instruction(s) *34* Anleitung

insulin *51* Insulin

insurance card *6* Versichertenkarte

intake *48* Zufuhr

interest *72* interessieren

interesting *11* interessant

intermediate diploma *11* Zwischenprüfung

intermediate French *74* Französisch auf fortgeschrittenem Anfängerniveau

internal *46T* innere/r/s

interpersonal skills *71* soziale Kompetenz

interval *59T* Abstand

interview sb *73* mit jdm ein Vorstellungsgespräch führen

interviewee *76* Befragte/r, Bewerber(in)

interviewer *76* Interviewer/in

introduce *53* einführen

introduction *53* Einführung

invasive *44* invasiv

invite *73* einladen

involve *42* mit sich bringen

involved in *11* beteiligt an

irregular *62* unregelmäßig

issue *47* Frage, Problem

item *35* Artikel

J

jacket *28* Jacke

jar *50* Glas

jaw *30* Kiefer

jealous *68* eifersüchtig, neidisch

jewellery *56* Schmuck

jigsaw *31* Puzzle

job interview *41* Vorstellungsgespräch

job opening *13* offene Stelle, Stellenangebot

join sb *37* sich jdm anschließen

joint *12* Gelenk

joy (of sth) *68* Freude (über etw)

juice *49* Saft

just *53* nur, gerade, bloß

K

keep: ~ **food down** *24* Nahrung bei sich behalten; ~ **records** *14* Aufzeichnungen führen, Akten halten; ~ **sb active** *61* jdn auf Trab halten

key *16T* Schlüssel

kick in *68* einsetzen

kidney *30* Niere

kind *17T* Art

kind of *54T* irgendwie

knee *30* Knie

knowledge *11* Wissen, Kenntnisse

known *57* bekannt

knuckle *30* (Finger-)Knöchel

L

label *15* Etikett; *16* beschriften; ~ **printer** *15* Etikettendrucker

laboratory/lab *12* Labor

lack *25* Mangel

largely *38* hauptsächlich, vor allem

last *56* dauern

latest *53* letzte/r/s, jüngste/r/s

laxative *32* Abführmittel

lazy *47T* faul

lead *51* führen

leader *72T* Leiter/in

leaflet *11* Broschüre, Merkblatt

leave out *34* weglassen

leave school *20* von der Schule abgehen

legally *13* gesetzlich, von Gesetzes wegen

length *11* Länge

lesson *31* Lehre, Lektion

letter of application *72* Bewerbungsschreiben

lettuce leaves *68* Salatblätter

level *38* Rate, Quote; *50* Spiegel

lie: ~ **around** *45* herumliegen; ~ **back** *56* sich auf den Rücken legen; ~ **down** *46T* sich hinlegen

life, lives *25* Leben

life-size *31* lebensgroß

lifestyle *51* Lebensweise, Lebensführung

life-threatening *42* lebensbedrohlich

light *27* leicht

likely *25* wahrscheinlich

limit *49T* begrenzen, beschränken

lip *21T* Lippe

live up to sth *63* einer Sache gerecht werden, etw erfüllen

liver *30* Leber

local *23* ortsansässig

local anaesthetic *27* örtliche Betäubung

lonely *47T* einsam

long *24T* lang; **as** ~ **as** *35T* solange

long-distance runner *61* Langstreckenläufer/in

look: ~ **after sb** *47* sich um jdn kümmern; ~ **forward to sth** *72* sich auf etw freuen; **have a** ~ *9* nachschauen

looks *62* Aussehen

lose weight *51* abnehmen

loud *56* laut

low *62* niedrig

lumbar puncture *61* Lumbalpunktion

lungs *21T* Lunge

M

machine *13* Gerät, Maschine

madness *68* Irrsinn

mainly *25* hauptsächlich

major *21T* Haupt-

majority *64* Mehrheit, größter Teil

make sth up *46* sich etw ausdenken, etw erfinden

make sure *47T* dafür sorgen

make use of *72T* nutzen

malnutrition *62T* Unterernährung

manage *7* schaffen, einrichten; *71* verwalten

manager *47T* Geschäftsführer/in

manner *13* Art (und Weise)

map *36* Karte, Plan

maple syrup *49* Ahornsirup

marital status *73* Familienstand

mark *53* markieren

marry *72* heiraten

mass *62* Masse

massage *44T* Massage; *44* massieren

match *7* zuordnen

material *11* Material

mature *11* hier: ältere

meal *33* Mahlzeit, Essen

mean *44T* bedeuten, heißen

measles *23* Masern

measure *20* messen

meat *49* Fleisch

medical *17* medizinisch, ärztlich

medical administration *11* medizinische Verwaltungsaufgaben

medical assistant *6* Medizinische Fachangestellte/r

medical attention *63* ärztliche Behandlung, ärztliche Hilfe

medical condition *31* Leiden, Beschwerden

medical consultation *31* medizinische Beratung

medical history *9* Krankengeschichte

medical practice *14* Arztpraxis

medical receptionist *11* Sprechstundenhilfe

medical supplies *14* Sanitätsartikel

medication *17T* Medikamente; *33* Medikation

medicine *17* Arzneimittel; *31* Medizin

meet (sb) *37* sich (mit jdm) treffen; **Nice to** ~ **you.** *56* Schön, Sie kennenzulernen.

meet expectations *65* Erwartungen erfüllen

meeting *13* Sitzung, Besprechung, Treffen

member *11* Mitglied

membership *71* Mitgliedschaft; ~ **organization** *71* Fachverband, Berufsverband

memo pad *15* Notizzettelblock

mental *40* geistig

mental illness *62* psychische Erkrankung

message *57* Botschaft, Nachricht

middle *21T* Mitte, mittlerer Teil

middle ear *21* Mittelohr

midwifery *71* Geburtshilfe

migraine *18* Migräne

mild *25* leicht

mile *20* Meile

milk: full fat ~ *50* Vollmilch; **skimmed** ~ *50* entrahmte/fettarme Milch; **whole** ~ *66* Vollmilch

mind *65* Verstand, Geist, Kopf; *67* (etwas) dagegen haben, ausmachen; **Never** ~. *23T* Macht nichts.

minor *35T* klein, gering

minority *34* Minderzahl

miserable *68* elend

miss sth *63* etw verpassen

miss out on sth *73* sich etw entgehen lassen

missing *10* fehlend

mistake *35* Fehler

mistakenly *38* fälschlich

mixed up *68* durcheinander, vertauscht

mix-up *35T* Durcheinander, Verwechslung

mobile phone *37* Handy

monitor *52T* überwachen

mood swing *63* Stimmungsschwankungen

motivate *73* motivieren

motivation *65* Motivation

mouse, mice *57* Maus, Mäuse

mouth *21* Mund

move *20* umziehen; *56* bewegen; ~ **sb** *31* (Patienten) verlegen; ~ **on to sth** *73* zu etw übergehen; ~ **house** 9 umziehen

movement 12 Bewegung

multiple sclerosis 56 Multiple Sklerose

muscle 18 Muskel

My goodness. 35T Meine Güte!

N

name 21 nennen, benennen

nasal passage 21 Nasengang

nasty 67 böse, schlimm

National Health Service 23 Nationaler Gesundheitsdienst

nationality 73 Staatsange-hörigkeit

nationally set 11 landesweit einheitlich

native speaker 74 Mutter-sprachler/in

naturally 49T von Natur aus

nausea 34 Übelkeit

near 18 nahe

neck 22 Hals, Nacken

need 40 Bedürfnis

need to do sth 9 etw tun müssen

needle-thread combination 26 Nadel-Faden-Kombination

negative 20 Verneinung

nerve 52T Nerv; ~ **cell** 57 Nervenzelle; ~-**racking** 77 nervenaufreibend

nervous 17T nervös

nervous system 57 Nerven-system

network 31 Netzwerk

neurologist 55 Neurologe/-in

Never mind. 23T Macht nichts.

Nice to meet you. 56 Schön, Sie kennenzulernen.

night school 71 Abendschule

noise 56 Geräusch

noisy 56 laut

non-nutritional foods 53 Lebensmittel ohne Nährwert

normally 40T normalerweise

nose 20 Nase

note 15 Notiz; 11 notieren, aufschreiben

notice 23T bemerken

nowadays 44 heutzutage

numb 61 (Gefühl:) taub

numbness 61 Taubheit

nurse 12 Krankenschwester/-pfleger

nursing home 71 Pflegeheim

nutrition 48 Ernährung

nutritional 63 Ernährungs-; **non-~ foods** 53 Lebensmittel ohne Nährwert

O

obese 48 fettleibig

obesity 62 Fettleibigkeit

obsess about sth 68 sich andauernd/zwanghaft mit etw beschäftigen

obsession 62 Besessenheit, Wahn, Zwang

occur 47 auftreten; 57 vorkommen

(the) odd one out 52 etwas, das nicht dazugehört

oesophagus 21 Oesophagus

offer 44 anbieten, bieten

office supplies 13 Bürobedarf

officially 66 offiziell

oil 49 Öl

ointment 35 Salbe, Wundsalbe

old fashioned 73 altmodisch

olfactory nerve 21 Geruchs-nerv

olive 49 Olive

on foot 36T zu Fuß

ongoing 31 laufend, andauernd

onion 49 Zwiebel

open 61 öffnen; **in the ~** 63 offen

opinion 11 Meinung, Ansicht

optician 36 Optiker

order 13 Reihenfolge; 35T Bestellung; 13 bestellen; **in ~ to** 9 um ... zu

organ 21T Organ

organize 71 organisieren

ossicles 21 Gehörknöchelchen

(the) other day 54T neulich

otherwise 34 anders

otoscope 26 Otoskop

out of date 73 veraltet, überholt

outer ear 21 Außenohr

outgoing 13 kontaktfreudig

outlook 61 Einstellung

outside 21 Außenseite; 47T außerhalb

overall 38 Gesamt-

overeat 62T zu viel essen, sich überfressen

overeating 62 übermäßiges Essen

over-the-counter 32 frei verkäuflich

overweight 25 übergewichtig

overworked 25 überarbeitet

P

packet 32 Packung

pad 56 Polster, Kissen

paediatrician 12 Kinderarzt/-ärztin

pain 8 Schmerz, Schmerzen; **be in ~** 8 Schmerzen haben

painful 20 schmerzhaft

painkiller 32 Schmerzmittel

painless 44T schmerzlos

palate 21 Gaumen

palm oil 49T Palmöl

paper clip 15 Büroklammer

paragraph 41 (Text:) Absatz

part 11 Teil; **in the ~ of** 25 auf Seiten der

part of the body 30 Körperteil

part time 11 Teilzeit-

partially 40 teilweise, zum Teil

particular 7T spezielle/r/s; **anything in ~** 49T etwas Besonderes

pass 11 (Prüfung) bestehen; **~ over sth** 21T hier: über etw streichen; **~ through** 50 hindurchgehen

passage 21T Gang, Weg

past 60 Vergangenheit

patient 8 Patient/in; 47 geduldig

patient record file 10 Patientenakte, Krankenakte

pay 77 Gehalt, Lohn, Bezahlung

payment 13 Zahlung

pedestrian subway 36 Fußgängerunterführung

pelvic examination 40 gynäkologische Untersuchung

per cent 25 Prozent

percentage 48 Anteil, Prozentsatz

perfectly 46 völlig

perhaps 57 vielleicht

period 59T Zeitraum, Zeitabschnitt; 68 Periode

permanent 68 dauernd

person: in ~ 11 persönlich

personal details 10 persönliche Angaben

personality 13 Persönlichkeit

personnel 13 Personal

pharmaceutical *16T* pharmazeutisch, Pharma-

pharmacist *32* Apotheker/in

pharmacy *32* Apotheke

phone call *7* Telefongespräch, Anruf

phone in *40T* anrufen

phrase *54* Redewendung, Ausdruck

physical *40* körperlich

physiotherapist *12* Physiotherapeut/in

physiotherapy *33* Physiotherapie

pick up *35T* abholen

picky *63* wählerisch

piece of equipment *26* Ausrüstungsgegenstand

pill *32* Pille

pilot trial *31* Pilotversuch, Pilotprojekt

pins and needles *54T* Kribbeln

place *36* Platz, Ort

plaster *28* Pflaster

play a part *64T* eine Rolle spielen

pleasant *37* angenehm

plenty of *22* viel(e)

plum *48* Pflaume

poem *39* Gedicht

poisoning *23* Vergiftung

police station *31* Polizeiwache

polite *13* höflich

politeness *6* Höflichkeit

poll *38* Umfrage

poor *41* schlecht, dürftig

pop *21* ploppen

popularity *53* Beliebtheit

population *63* Bevölkerung

pork *49T* Schwein(efleisch)

possible *44T* möglich

possibly *57* möglicherweise

postcode *9* Postleitzahl

post-graduate diploma *72T* weiterführender Studienabschluss

power *65* Kraft, Macht

practice *8* Übung, Training; *9* Praxis

Practice makes perfect. *76T* Übung macht den Meister.

practise *9* üben

precaution *38* Vorkehrung, Vorsichtsmaßnahme

predict *59T* voraussagen

prefer *7T* vorziehen, (lieber) mögen

pregnancy *49* Schwangerschaft

pregnant *17* schwanger

preparation *76T* Vorbereitung

prepare *39* (sich) vorbereiten; *50* (Essen) kochen, zubereiten

prescribe *22* verschreiben, verordnen

prescription *8* Rezept

prescription medication *40* verschreibungspflichtige Medikamente

present *74* Gegenwart; *13* anwesend, zugegen; *75* gegenwärtig, aktuell; *31* zeigen, präsentieren

presentation *39* Präsentation

presenter *68* Moderator/in

pressure *13* Druck

pretty *23T* hübsch; *72T* ziemlich

prevent *38* verhüten, verhindern

previous *72* vorhergehend, vorig

primarily *63* zu(aller)erst

Primary-progressive MS *59* Primär-progrediente MS

print *15* ausdrucken

printer *15* Drucker

privacy *13* Privatsphäre

probably *22* wahrscheinlich

procedure *27* Vorgang, Verfahren(sweise); *46* Eingriff

produce *51* herstellen, erstellen

professional *71* beruflich

professional association *73* Berufsverband

progress *44T* Fortschritt

progress *57* Verlauf; *59* verlaufen

progressive *52T* fortschreitend, progressiv

Progressive-relapsing MS *59* Schubförmig-progrediente MS

promise *35T* versprechen

properly *44T* richtig, ordentlich

pros and cons *53* Pro und Contra

protect *26* schützen

protein *57* Protein

prove *57* beweisen, nachweisen

provide *13* bieten

provider *47* Anbieter

psychological *63* psychologisch

public *13* Publikum; *38* öffentlich

pull *39* ziehen

pulse *25* Puls; **take sb's ~** *25* jds Puls messen

pump *35* Pumpe

purge *65* kontrolliertes Vomitieren, Erbrechen

purging (controlled vomiting) *62* kontrolliertes Erbrechen

pushchair *40* Buggy *(Kinderwagen)*

pushy: be ~ *63* zudringlich sein, übermäßig ehrgeizig sein

put sb at risk *51* jdn einem Risiko aussetzen

Q

qualification *11* Abschluss, Qualifikation, Voraussetzung

qualified *13* ausgebildet, qualifiziert

quarter: a ~ past *7* Viertel nach; **a ~ to** *7* Viertel vor

questionnaire *17* Fragebogen

quite *25* ziemlich

R

race *57* Rasse

radio frequency *55* Funkwellenlänge

radiologist *12* Radiologe/-in

range *71* Reihe, Auswahl

rank *13* einstufen

rapeseed *(BE)*, **canola** *(AE)* *49* Raps

rash *23T* Ausschlag

rate *38* Quote, Rate; *41* einstufen

rather than *53* statt

reach *36T* erreichen

react *47T* reagieren

reaction *17* Reaktion

reader *73* Leser/in

ready for business *13* betriebsbereit

reality *69* Wirklichkeit

reason *25* Grund; **for no ~** *68* ohne Grund

reassurance *44* Beruhigung

reassure sb *27* jdn beruhigen

receipt *6* Quittung, Beleg

receive *9* erhalten, bekommen

recent *48* aktuell, jüngere/r/s, letzte/r/s; **in ~ years** *38* in den letzten Jahren

recently *24T* in letzter Zeit

reception *6* Anmeldung, Rezeption

reckon *48* schätzen

recognise *25* erkennen

recognized *60* anerkannt

recommend *49T* empfehlen

recommendation *76* Empfehlung

record *68* aufnehmen, *hier:* filmen

records *14* Aufzeichnungen, Unterlagen

reduce *47T* verringern

refer to sth *38* sich auf etw beziehen

reference *73* Referenz, Zeugnis

register sb *13* jdn registrieren, aufnehmen; **~ with sb** *9* sich (bei jdm) anmelden

registered *71* registriert

regular *18* regelmäßig

relapse *59T* Schub

Relapsing-remitting MS *59* Schubförmig-remittierende MS

relationship *47* Verhältnis, Beziehung

relative *11* Verwandte/r

relax *27* sich entspannen

relaxed *44* locker, entspannt

relaxing *44* entspannend

relaxing bath *76* Entspannungsbad

relevant to *73* relevant für, wichtig für

reliable *70* zuverlässig

relieve *44T* lindern, abbauen

rely on sth *47T* auf etw angewiesen sein

remember *21T* denken an, nicht vergessen; *24T* sich erinnern

remission *59T* Abklingen, Remission

remote *31* fern, Fern-

remove *54T* (Kleidung) ausziehen

renew *40T* erneuern

repair *18* reparieren

replace *66* ersetzen

reply n *75* Antwort

report *38* Bericht; *53* berichten

represent *73* darstellen, repräsentieren

require *71* benötigen, erfordern, verlangen, voraussetzen

required *11* erforderlich, nötig

requirement *73* Anforderung, Bedürfnis

research *38* Forschung, Untersuchungen

research sth *61* sich über etw erkundigen

researcher *57* Forscher/in, Wissenschaftler/in

resonance *55* Resonanz

respect *13* respektieren

respond *66* reagieren, *(auf eine Behandlung)* ansprechen

response *6* Antwort; *27* Reaktion

responsibility *73* Verantwortlichkeit, Zuständigkeit

responsible *70* verantwortungsbewusst; **~ for** *71* verantwortlich, zuständig für

rest *22* Ruhe; *51* Rest

rest (with sth) *73* (auf etw) ruhen

rest home *47* Seniorenheim

result *8* Ergebnis, Resultat

retail *77* Einzelhandel

retire *61* sich zur Ruhe setzen

retirement *47* Ruhestand

return *27* zurückkehren, wiederkommen

rich (in) *50* reich (an)

right away *46T* sofort

rise *38* Anstieg, Zunahme; *38* ansteigen

risk *42* Risiko; *68* riskieren

risky *43* riskant

role-play *76* Rollenspiel; *10* mit verteilten Rollen spielen

roll up *24T* *(Ärmel)* hochkrempeln

roof *21T* Dach

routine test *18* Routineuntersuchung

rower *51* Ruderer/-in

rude *70* unhöflich, unverschämt

rule sth out *59T* etw ausschließen

rump *39* Rumpf

run sth *31* etw leiten, führen

rush around *47T* umherhetzen

rushed *44T* gehetzt

S

safe *31* sicher

sales area *74* Verkaufsfläche

sales target *72* Umsatzziel, Verkaufsziel

saline *35* Salz-; **~ infusion** *35* Kochsalzlösung

salmon *49* Lachs

sandwich release (course) *74* Kurs mit abwechselnder theoretischer und praktischer Ausbildung

satisfy requirements *11* Bedingungen erfüllen

saturated *50* gesättigt

sausage *49* (Brat-)Wurst

say: have your ~ in sth *77* seine Meinung zu etw äußern

scalpel *26* Skalpell

scare *43* Schrecken

scare sb *42* jdm Angst einjagen, jdn erschrecken

scared: be ~ of sth *41* vor etw Angst haben

scary *40T* unheimlich

scheme *11* Programm, Projekt, Plan

school: ~ dinner *53* Schulessen; **~ gates** *53* Schultor; **~ leaver** *11* Schulabgänger/in

scientific *48* wissenschaftlich

scissors *15* Schere

Scotland *31* Schottland

scratch *24* Kratzer, Kratzwunde

screwdriver *24T* Schraubenzieher

seat: take a ~ *6* Platz nehmen

Secondary-progressive MS *59* Sekundär-progrediente MS

secretarial *72T* Sekretariats-

secretary *61* Sekretär/in

section break *73* Abschnittswechsel

seem *22* scheinen

self-care *52T* Eigenfürsorge

self-esteem *47T* Selbstwertgefühl

self-image *65* Selbstbild

self-respect *47T* Selbstachtung

self-study *71* Selbststudium

semi-circular canals *21* Bogengänge

send *15* (ver)senden, (ver)schicken

senior *23* älter, ranghöher

sensation *54* Gefühl, Empfindung

sense *43* Sinn

sensible *76T* vernünftig

sensitive to sth *63* auf etw Rücksicht nehmen, einfühlsam sein

separate *21* trennen; *59T* einzeln, getrennt

serious *35T* schwer, ernst

serve *53* servieren; ~ **sb** *35* jdn bedienen

service *13* Dienst, Dienstleistung

setup *31* Aufbau, Anordnung, Einrichtung

set up *31* einrichten, aufbauen

several *35T* einige, mehrere

severe *25* *(Schmerzen:)* heftig

sexual *38* sexuell

sheet *42* Blatt (Papier)

shin *30* Schienbein

shipment *35* Sendung, Lieferung

shop assistant *33* Verkäufer/in

short of breath *55* außer Atem

shoulder *23T* Schulter

show *16T* zeigen

shy *23T* schüchtern

sick *39* krank

sick note *22* Krankschreibung, Attest

sickness *62* Übelkeit

side effect *33* Nebenwirkung

sight *28T* Anblick

sign *16T* unterschreiben

similar *9* ähnlich

since *38* seit

sincerely: Yours ~ *72* *(Brief:)* Mit freundlichen Grüßen

sit down *23T* sich (hin)setzen

size *62T* Größe

sketch *36* Skizze

skills *11* Fertigkeiten, Fähigkeiten

skimmed milk *50* entrahmte/ fettarme Milch

skin *26* Haut

skinny *68* mager, dürr

skip *25* Aussetzer, Unregelmäßigkeit

skydiving *76* Fallschirmspringen

sleeping tablet *32* Schlaftablette

sleeve *24T* Ärmel

slim *68* schlank

slip *24T* abrutschen

slow (down) *57* verlangsamen

smallpox *40* Pocken

smart *71* intelligent, aufgeweckt; *76T* *(Kleidung:)* schick

smear test *18* Abstrich

smell *21T* Geruch

smell (of sth) *42* (nach etw) riechen

smelly *43* stinkend

smoke *25* rauchen

smoker *49T* Raucher/in

sneeze *23T* niesen

soccer *(AE)* *64T* Fußball

society *61* Gesellschaft

solve *47* lösen

soon enough *62T* früh genug

sore *22* wund

sore throat *22* Halsschmerzen

sound *37T* klingen

sound wave *21* Schallwelle

South African *60* südafrikanisch, aus Südafrika

special *31* speziell, besonders

specialist *18* Facharzt/-ärztin; ~ **register** *23* Facharztregister

specialize *12* sich spezialisieren

specific *73* konkret, genau

specified *71* festgelegt

speculum *43* Spekulum

spell *8* buchstabieren

spelling *8* Schreibweise

spend *44* *(Zeit)* verbringen

spending *64T* Ausgaben, Etat

spinach *49T* Spinat

spleen *30* Milz

splinter *26* Splitter

spot *23T* Punkt, Fleck; *62T* erkennen; *69* entdecken

sprain *26* Verstauchung

spread *38* Ausbreitung; *40T* verbreiten

square *62* Quadrat

staff *11* Personal

staff appraisal *73* Mitarbeiterbeurteilung

staffroom *12* Personalraum

stage *31* Phase, Abschnitt; *59T* Stadium

stairs *16* Treppe

stamp *15* stempeln

stand *37* stehen; *70* ertragen

standard *71* Anforderung, Richtlinie, Norm

stapler *15* Heftgerät, Tacker

starting point *36* Ausgangspunkt

starvation *68* Hungern, Unterernährung

starve oneself *65* hungern; ~ **sb/sth of sth** *62T* jdm/etw etw vorenthalten

state *13* Staat, Land

statement *6* Aussage, Behauptung

statistics *63* Statistik(en)

stay *25* bleiben

steady *59T* stetig, gleichmäßig

step *27* Schritt; **take ~s** *63* Schritte unternehmen

sterilization *12* Sterilisation

stethoscope *26* Stethoskop

still *20* (immer) noch; *52* trotzdem, dennoch

sting *27T* schmerzen, brennen

stirrup *21* Steigbügel

stitch *24T* Stich; *24* nähen; **take out ~es** *27* Fäden ziehen

stock levels *74* Lagerbestände

stomach *21T* Magen; ~ **complaints** *34* Magenbeschwerden

stone *55* Stein

store *15* lagern

storeroom *16* Lagerraum

straight away *18* sofort

straight on *16* geradeaus

strange *54T* seltsam

strength *73* Stärke

stressed *25* gestresst; ~-**out** *25* gestresst

stressful *76T* anstrengend, stressig

strike *60* zuschlagen

study *11* Studium, Ausbildung; *48* Untersuchung, Studie; *23* studieren; untersuchen; ~ **for sth** *11* für etw lernen

stuff: ... and ~ *72T* und so

stupid *62* töricht, doof

subject *73* (Schul-, Studien-) Fach

substance *50* Stoff, Substanz

subtype *59* Subtyp, Untertyp

succeed *31* Erfolg haben, erfolgreich sein

success *47T* Erfolg

suffer from sth *25* an etw leiden

sufferer *38* Erkrankte/r, Patient/in

sugared pill *33* Dragee

sugary *51* süß, zuckerhaltig

suggest *38* hinweisen auf, hindeuten auf

suggestion *40* Vorschlag

suitable *11* geeignet

summarize *11* zusammenfassen

summary *31* Zusammenfassung

sunny *37* sonnig

suntan lotion *32* Sonnenmilch

supplies *14* Artikel, Bedarf, Vorräte

support *63* Unterstützung, Hilfe; ~ **centre** *61* Hilfszentrum; ~ **organization** *47* Hilfsorganisation

supportive *13* hilfreich, verständnisvoll; *61* verständnisvoll

suppose *44T* annehmen, glauben

sure *18* sicher

surely *64T* sicher(lich), bestimmt

surgery *6* (Arzt-)Praxis; ~ **charge** *6* Praxisgebühr

surgical needle-holder *26* Operationsnadelhalter

surprising *73* überraschend

suspended pocket file *15* Hängesammler, Hängeregister

swab *22* Tupfer; Abstrich

swallow *21T* schlucken

sweet: have a ~ tooth *49T* eine Vorliebe für Süßes haben

sweeten *49* süßen

swollen *22* geschwollen

sympathetic *27* mitfühlend, verständnisvoll

sympathy *67* Mitgefühl, Mitleid, Verständnis

symptom *18* Symptom

syringe *18* (Ohr etc.) ausspülen

T

tablet *17* Tablette

take: ~ in (air) *21T* (Luft) einatmen; ~ **off** *28* (Kleidung) ausziehen; ~ **off** *31* durchstarten, sich verbreiten; ~ **part in sth** *13* an etw teilnehmen

take a seat *6* Platz nehmen

take blood *28* Blut abnehmen

take blood pressure *29* den Blutdruck messen

take care of sb *47T* auf jdn aufpassen, sich um jdn kümmern

take effect *27* wirken, Wirkung zeigen

take one's temperature *22* bei jdm Fieber messen

take sb's pulse *25* jds Puls messen

take steps *63* Schritte unternehmen

take time off *47T* sich freinehmen, sich Zeit nehmen

take X-rays *12* röntgen

take out stitches *27* Fäden ziehen

take (it in) turns *24* sich abwechseln

take your life *65* sich umbringen

talk *47* Vortrag

talkative *70* gesprächig

target *71* Ziel, Zielvorgabe

task *47T* Aufgabe

taste *21T* Geschmack; *21T* schmecken

teaspoonful *32T* Teelöffel

technical *73* technisch, Fach-

technician *60* Techniker/in

technology *31* Technik, Technologie

temperature *23T* Fieber; **take one's ~** *22* bei jdm Fieber messen

temping agency *72T* Zeitarbeitsfirma

temporary *72T* vorübergehend, (Arbeit:) befristet

tend *25* dazu neigen

tense *41* angespannt

terrible *23T* fürchterlich

therapy *63* Therapie

therefore *73* daher

thermometer *22* Thermometer

thigh *30* Oberschenkel

thin *62* dünn

thinness *68* Schlankheit

thought *63* Gedanke, Überlegung

throat *20* Rachen, Hals

tie off stitches *27* Fäden verknoten

tight *28* eng, fest

till *35T* bis

time: take ~ off *47T* sich freinehmen, sich Zeit nehmen

tin *35* Dose

tingling *54T* Kribbeln

tiny *21* winzig

tired *22* müde

together (with) *21T* zusammen (mit)

tongue *21* Zunge

tonsillitis *22* Mandelentzündung

tonsils *22* Mandeln

tooth, teeth *21T* Zahn, Zähne; **have a sweet ~** *49T* eine Vorliebe für Süßes haben

tourniquet *26* Venenstauer

trachea *21* Trachea

traditional *41* traditionell

traffic *76T* (Straßen-)Verkehr

train *13* ausbilden; ~ **as** *47* eine Ausbildung machen zum/r

trainee *21* Auszubildende/r

trainer *76* Ausbilder/in

training *11* Ausbildung

transfer *57* Übermittlung; *73* übertragen

translate *17* übersetzen

transmit *38* übertragen

traumatic *63* traumatisch

tray *20* Schale

treat *12* behandeln

treatment room *12* Behandlungszimmer

trial *31* Test

trouble *22* Schwierigkeit(en), Problem(e)

true *6* wahr

trust *38* Stiftung; *47T* Vertrauen

trust sb *44T* jdm vertrauen

try *24T* versuchen

tube *21T* Röhre

tummy *68* Bauch

turn: ~ sth into sth *21* etw in etw umwandeln; ~ **left/ right** *16T* links/rechts abbiegen; ~ **off** *13* ab-/ausschalten; ~ **to sth** *63* sich einer Sache zuwenden; **take (it in) ~s** *24* sich abwechseln

TV programme *53* Fernsehsendung; **TV show** *53* Fernsehsendung

tweezers *26* Pinzette

type *51* Typ

typewriter *73* Schreibmaschine

typical *12* typisch

U

unable *64* unfähig

unattractive *68* unattraktiv

uncomfortable: feel ~ *41* sich unwohl fühlen

uncommon *59T* selten, ungewöhnlich

uncontrolled *63* unkontrolliert

undergo *61* sich unterziehen, durchmachen

understanding *47T* verständnisvoll

underweight *66* untergewichtig

undress *40* sich ausziehen

unfortunately *35* leider

unfriendly *42* unfreundlich

unhealthy *64* krankhaft

unit *66* Einheit

unless *34* wenn nicht

unplug sth *13* den Stecker von etw herausziehen

unsweetened *49* ungesüßt

until *36* bis

unusual *37* ungewöhnlich, außergewöhnlich

urine sample *33* Urinprobe

Uruguayan *68* aus Uruguay

use *31* Gebrauch

useful *44* nützlich, geeignet

usually *14* normalerweise, gewöhnlich

V

vaccination *46* Impfung

vaccine *32T* Impfstoff

van *53* Lieferwagen

varied *61* verschieden(artig), abwechslungsreich

vegetable oil *50* Pflanzenöl

versatile *73* vielseitig

victory *53* Sieg

video conferencing *31* Videokonferenz

view *25* Ansicht

viewer *53* Zuschauer/in

village *20* Dorf

violinist *41* Geiger/in

virus *38* Virus

vision *54T* Sehen, Sehkraft

visit *20* Besuch; *14* besuchen

visitor *17* Besucher/in

vocational qualification *71* Berufsabschluss

volunteer *31* sich zur Verfügung stellen

vomit *23T* sich erbrechen

W

waiting room *6* Wartezimmer

wake up *61* aufwachen

wake-up call *25* Weckruf

warmth *47T* Wärme

warn *32* warnen, darauf hinweisen

warning sign *25* Warnsignal

watch *56* Armbanduhr

watch TV *44* fernsehen

way *21T* Art (und Weise)

(ear) wax *18* Ohrenschmalz

weak *25* schwach

weakness *47T* Schwäche

weather *37* Wetter

weigh *63* abwiegen, wiegen

weight *62* Gewicht; **~ loss** *62T* Gewichtsverlust, -abnahme

weird *54T* seltsam, unheimlich

welcome: You're ~. *6* Bitte. Gern geschehen.

well: as ~ *72T* auch; **~-organized** *70* gut organisiert

what life has to throw at sb *61* *etwa:* was das Leben einem zu bieten hat

wheelchair *40* Rollstuhl

whether *31* ob

whiplash *55* Schleudertrauma

whole *31* ganz

whole milk *66* Vollmilch

wide *22* weit

widespread *38* weit verbreitet

windpipe *21* Luftröhre

within *11* innerhalb

wonder *64T* sich fragen

wonderful *27* wunderbar

wooden stick *46T* Holzstab

wordfield *51* Wortfeld

work experience *11* Berufs-/ Arbeitserfahrung; **~ routine** *71* Arbeitsablauf

work overtime *70* Überstunden machen

work-based assignment *11* praktische Prüfungsaufgabe

working day *13* Arbeitstag

World Health Organization (WHO) *68* Weltgesundheitsorganisation

worried *41* besorgt, beunruhigt

worry: ~ about sth *54* sich um etw Sorgen machen; **Don't ~.** *6* Keine Sorge.

would rather (not) do sth *42* würden etwas lieber (nicht) tun

wrist *30* Handgelenk

writing: in ~ *71* schriftlich

written *11* schriftlich

X, Y

X-rays *12* Röntgenstrahlen; **take ~** *12* röntgen

Yours sincerely *72* *(Brief:)* Mit freundlichen Grüßen

Quellenverzeichnis

RF-Fotos
Alamy: S. 12/TetraImages, S. 14/3/Stockbroker, S. 18/1/TLF Design, S. 18/4/J. Nieuwnhuize,
   S. 18/6/A. Ross, S. 35/A. Rodriguez, S. 36/1(WV), S. 36/4(WV), S. 43/1/D. Green,
   S. 43/3/K. Sriskandan, S. 70/TetraImages, S. 72/1/2/ImageSource/E 056;
Corbis: S. 18/J. Justice (WV);
CV-Archiv: S. 43/4, S. 52;
IStockphoto: S. 37/1/2/5/6, S. 50;
V. Maly: S. 32/1;
Shutterstock: S. 18/3, S. 23/1/2/3/5, S. 37/3/4, S. 40/2, S. 45/3/4/5/7, S. 48/1/2

RM-Fotos
Alamy: S. 12/J. West, S. 12/T. del Amo, S. 12/J. Tack, S. 14/2/J. Wiedel, S. 17/Custom Medical Stock
   Photo, S. 18/2/blickwinkel, S. 20/2/F1online, S. 22/G. Palmer, S. 23/HBSS, S. 38/D. Crossland,
   S. 42/C. Pefley, S. 43/2/J. Hiebaum, S. 67/T. Manley, S. 72/2/Kolvenbach, S. 72/4/D. Frazier,
   S. 75/Aberystwyth, S. 77/ICP;
Corbis: S. 53/P. Dench;
Fotofinder: S. 6/1/Das Fotoarchiv/K. Rose, S. 6/2/Argus/Scholz(WV), S. 14/Blickwinkel/McPhoto,
   S. 20/1/Keystone/J. Zick, S. 31/1/Kurt Fuchs Presse Foto Design, S. 31/2/Blickwinkel/McPhoto,
   S. 32/2/Bildagentur-online, S. 40/3/allesalltag, S. 40/5/Photothek (WV), S. 41/Fotex/R. Zorn,
   S. 45/1/Stock4B/K. Blaschke, S. 45/2/Okapia, S. 46/images.de/W. Kunz, S. 47/Bildmaschine,
   S. 51/A1PIX, S. 54/Blickwinkel/McPhoto, S. 61/R. Weisflog, S. 65/S. Boness, S. 70/2/Westend61,
   S. 70/3/Stock4B/K. Blaschke;
Photoshot: S. 41/Zeng Yi;
Picture Alliance: S. 41/T. Shemetov, S. 45/6/Chromorange, S. 62/1/K. Brooks, S. 62/2/AJG,
   S. 63/Abaca Motte, S. 69/EPA efe Pereyra;
RiaNovosti: S. 19;

Cartoons
S. 39/Pete Oldham, S. 52/Mike Baldwin, CartoonStock: S. 76, S. 43